THE VITAMIN CURE

for Alcoholism

Orthomolecular Treatment of Addictions

ABRAM HOFFER, MD, PhD
AND ANDREW W. SAUL, PhD

Basic Health
PUBLICATIONS, INC.

The information contained in this book is based upon the research and personal and professional experiences of the authors. It is not intended as a substitute for consulting with your physician or other healthcare provider. Any attempt to diagnose and treat an illness should be done under the direction of a healthcare professional.

The publisher does not advocate the use of any particular healthcare protocol but believes the information in this book should be available to the public. The publisher and authors are not responsible for any adverse effects or consequences resulting from the use of the suggestions, preparations, or procedures discussed in this book. Should the reader have any questions concerning the appropriateness of any procedures or preparation mentioned, the authors and the publisher strongly suggest consulting a professional healthcare advisor.

Basic Health Publications, Inc.
28812 Top of the World Drive
Laguna Beach, CA 92651
949-715-7327 • www.basichealthpub.com

Library of Congress Cataloging-in-Publication Data

Hoffer, Abram
    The vitamin cure for alcoholism : orthomolecular treatment of addictions / Abram Hoffer and Andrew W. Saul.
        p. cm.
    Includes bibliographical references and index.
    ISBN 978-1-59120-254-7
    1. Alcoholism. 2. Alcoholism—Treatment. 3. Orthomolecular therapy.
I. Saul, Andrew W. II. Title.

    RC565.H624 2009
    362.292—dc22

                                                    2008054330

Editor: John Anderson
Typesetting/Book design: Gary A. Rosenberg
Cover design: Mike Stromberg

Printed in the United States of America

10   9   8   7   6   5   4   3   2   1

CONTENTS

ACKNOWLEDGMENTS

To Bill W., cofounder of Alcoholics Anonymous (AA), and to the three physicians—David Hawkins, Ed Boyle, and Russell Smith—who confirmed Bill's conclusion that alcoholics need to become well, and not merely abstinent. Bill was a seer with a vision and was therefore able to act in spite of negative pressure. Most of AA thought that vitamin therapy was none of his business, nor theirs. Bill W. knew that it was his business to help all alcoholics and other addicts not only be free of their addiction but to be comfortable with their new state of well-being and freedom.

—Abram Hoffer

I add my thanks to all the physicians and researchers who, in the face of medical opposition, have so ably demonstrated that high-dose vitamin therapy works. Some day soon, healthcare without megavitamin therapy will be seen as we today see childbirth without sanitation, or surgery without anesthetic. I dedicate this book to Colleen, who, in seeing that so clearly, helps me stay the course.

—Andrew W. Saul

FOREWORD

The prevalence of alcoholism reflects a fundamental ignorance or carelessness about nutrition, because the development of alcoholism generally requires years of heavy drinking. Prolonged consumption of large amounts of calories from alcoholic beverages, and other nonwhole foods such as refined sugar, is simply inconsistent with the rules of good nutrition, even if alcoholism and other addictions did not exist.

But they do. Therefore, this book can be a godsend for many persons—for those who suffer from alcohol addiction, for their friends and loved ones, and for those in the relevant helping professions. Its central message is that alcoholism is primarily a metabolic disease that should be treated with due consideration of its physiological roots. The old moralistic approach and the more recent behavioral and psychological treatment approaches have a dismal record of failure, largely because they pay little or no attention to the crucial physiological and nutritional needs of alcoholics.

The keys to more appropriate and effective approaches come from studies and from metabolic tests showing that alcoholism is a complex genetic-biochemical disorder more closely related to diabetes or to sugar metabolic syndrome than to any behavioral or psychological disorder. Although scientists widely agree that susceptibility to alcoholism is inherited (by roughly 10 percent of the population), treatment and support programs generally ignore this fact and its physiological implications. Likewise, malnutrition is well-known to physicians treating alcoholics, but they nearly always assume that malnutrition is a simple, predictable *consequence* of heavy drinking, not a complex, contributing *cause* of alcohol addiction. Nutrition is certainly not seen as the effective treatment it is.

My late mentor at the University of Texas, Roger J. Williams, devoted three books and over two dozen scientific articles to the problem of alcoholism. His work was remarkably advanced and insightful. Nearly fifty years ago, in his second book on alcoholism, *Alcoholism: The Nutritional Approach,* he summarized part of his work in animals: "Our first important finding is that [laboratory] rats exhibit a high degree of individuality in their behavior when they are all fed alike and treated alike in every way. . . . Our second finding is that this individuality in drinking behavior . . . is genetically determined. . . . A third finding [is that] what the rats have to eat, that is, the chemical composition of their food, is a potent factor in determining how great is their physiological urge to drink alcohol." Another of my senior colleagues at the University of Texas, William Shive, reported in 1955 that the amino acid L-glutamine protects bacterial cells from the toxic effects of alcohol. Dr. Williams and his coworkers soon found that poorly nourished rats decreased their voluntary consumption of alcohol by about 40 percent, on average, when L-glutamine was added to their diets. Later, they also found evidence that it is highly effective for some humans in reducing their appetite for alcohol.

Abram Hoffer and Andrew Saul have found that Dr. Williams's observations apply well to humans: vitamins and other nutritional factors play a potent role in countering the compulsion to drink. No treatment and no amount of social support is likely to achieve long-term abstinence without addressing these underlying biochemical issues.

Over the years, a few other researchers, practitioners, and laypersons have advocated similar ideas about alcohol and some other addictions. Unfortunately, these advocates have not yet found a sufficient audience to achieve a wide impact. There are several contributing reasons why this is so. Pharmaceutical companies have no financial incentive to research natural, unpatentable approaches to addiction. More fundamentally, such low-technology approaches have never become fashionable among medical researchers. Remarkably, the American Psychiatric Association and physicians in general recognize their limited ability to deal adequately with alcoholism by referring sufferers to a *lay* support organization, Alcoholics Anonymous (AA). Unfortunately, AA has limited itself by sidestepping nutrition. It didn't have to happen this way, as Drs. Hoffer and Saul explain. The cofounder of AA, Bill W., was treated by Dr. Hoffer in 1958 and into the 1960s. Bill found great benefit from a nutritional approach, repeated his success among many of his friends and associates, and despite great efforts, he was unable to influence the organization toward broadening its approach.

Human nature can be disheartening at times, especially in the face of such devastating problems as alcohol and drug addictions. The good news for readers of this book is that it offers "new" approaches and hope that you are unlikely to learn about elsewhere. When will the medical and other helping professions give serious consideration to these insights from genetics, human physiology, animal studies, the cofounder of AA, and a few pioneering researchers and physicians? I hope this book will hasten that time, by bringing relief and renewed health to legions of sufferers and also by nurturing so many successful advocates for advancement that their voices will finally become irresistible.

—Donald R. Davis, Ph.D.
Austin, Texas

CHAPTER 1

NUTRITIONAL FACTORS FOR ALCOHOLISM

Edith had been drinking up to 40 ounces of whiskey daily for three weeks. Her gait was unsteady, her speech was limited to a few words, she trembled and complained of jitters. She was admitted to the hospital and immediately given 400 milligrams of niacin intravenously, plus 3,000 mg of niacin and 2,000 mg of vitamin C by mouth. Within minutes, she had calmed down. The second day, she was given niacin (3,000 mg) and vitamin C (2,000 mg) after each meal. On the second morning she was still jittery, but by that afternoon she was well and remained so for the rest of her hospital stay.

Fred had been drinking for sixteen years and suffered three bouts of delirium tremens (DTs) with hallucinations. He was irritable and tense. He was given 2,000 mg of niacin and 2,000 mg of vitamin C after each of three meals. The same day, by 10:30 P.M., he was cooperative, pleasant, and related normally to others. He remained well in the hospital and after his discharge.

Neither of the above patients had responded to the medication in use for their condition. Both recovered on vitamin therapy. And that is what this book is about.

NOT A DISEASE

Nutrition can cure alcohol addiction. Alcoholism is not a disease, even though it has been so considered for many years. A person

1

called an "alcoholic" is an individual with a sick body who seeks relief and comfort by consuming alcohol in the same way that people seek help from aspirin, or eat too much sugar, or are given medication for their discomfort. Alcohol is a self-selected treatment. The individual has discovered through the years that alcohol provides more comfort than any other drug, and it is readily available and acceptable (within certain boundaries) by society. In time, that individual is sick not only from the original disorder but also from the ravages of the drinking itself.

So why do we call it alcoholism? Do we call a diabetic who has to take insulin an insulinic, or a person who has to take steroids for Addison's disease a steroidic, or an arthritic who takes aspirin to control pain an aspirinic? The term *alcoholic* is totally illogical and indefensible, even though it was helpful as long as there was little information about the real factors that lead to excessive drinking and to all addictions.

The real problem is that the alcoholic to be (we still have to use the term as there is no useful replacement) is not well. None of the common medical tests will show where the problem is as it is a case of severe malnutrition—not of calories but of the nutrients that are essential to properly metabolize food. Ever since working closely with Bill W. (Bill Wilson), cofounder of Alcoholics Anonymous (AA), I (A.H.) have thought that a person who is really well will not become an alcoholic. It doesn't mean he or she will not drink; rather, it means that like most of the population, they will use alcohol on occasion and not to the detriment of themselves, their families, and society. This idea first began to take shape when research in the 1950s on the therapeutic effect of vitamin B_3 (niacin or niacinamide) with schizophrenic patients showed that patients with the double diagnosis of alcoholism and schizophrenia could not recover until they were treated with optimum (meaning large) doses of B_3.

Bill understood this perfectly, for even after he had been abstinent for many years, he was still not well. He suffered from immense anxiety, tension, and fatigue, but in spite of what should have been disabling, he was able to function. After he started taking niacin (3,000 mg daily for two weeks), his symptoms vanished and he remained free of them. He was determined to give as many members of AA as possible the benefit of the same vitamin. Without telling me, he conducted a trial of niacin on thirty friends and colleagues in New York. Most of them were very

WHO WAS BILL W.?

"Bill Wilson is the greatest social architect of the 20th century."
—ALDOUS HUXLEY

Bill W. (William Griffith Wilson, 1895–1971), the man who would cofound Alcoholics Anonymous (AA), was born to a hard-drinking household in rural Vermont. When he was ten, his parents split up and Bill was raised by his maternal grandparents. He served in the army in World War One, and although not seeing combat, Bill had more than ample opportunities to drink. In the 1920s, he achieved considerable success as an inside trader on Wall Street, but a combination of drunkenness and the stock market crash of 1929 drained what was left of his fortune and his capability to enjoy life.

Hard knocks, a religious experience, and a growing sense that by helping other alcoholics he could best help himself led Bill to create one of the world's most famous introductions: "My name is Bill W., and I'm an alcoholic." Even as Alcoholics Anonymous slowly grew, many of Bill's financial and personal problems endured, most notably depression. Dr. Hoffer introduced Bill to the concept of megavitamin therapy. After he took niacin for a few weeks, Bill's fatigue and depression, which had plagued him for years, were gone. Bill then wrote "The Vitamin B_3 Therapy" and thousands of copies of this extraordinary pamphlet were distributed, although it made Bill unpopular with the medical members of the board of AA International.

productive and sober members of AA, but they all suffered from the common affliction of alcoholics even when they are not drinking. After three months, he showed me his data:

- After one month, ten were well.

- After the second month, another ten had recovered.

- The rest had shown no improvement after the third month.

By this time, I had also treated a number of alcoholics and had seen similar recoveries.

Interest in the role of vitamins as treatment inevitably drew my attention to the problem of hypoglycemia (low blood sugar). This became the infamous "H word" for the medical establishment, but it is a real condition and is now given a different name and is often diagnosed as type 2 diabetes. I tested over 300 alcoholics with a glucose tolerance test and did not find even one patient who had a normal result. The treatment was to avoid sugar, which is very difficult, especially for alcoholics. Alcohol, a very simple carbohydrate, is basically a liquid sugar and is at least as harmful to health as sugar. Addiction to sugar starts during childhood and later becomes the more sophisticated form of addiction to the alcohol.

This book outlines the nutritional factors that have been shown to be successful in treating alcoholism and depression. When alcoholics are able to abstain from alcohol on their own, this is the course to follow. Some of them can even become social drinkers on a very small scale, but not many. However, if started on this nutritional program very early, many more could achieve normalcy. I know of many alcoholics who did not want to stop drinking, but did agree to take niacin. Over the years, they gradually were able to reduce their alcohol intake until they brought it under control. I suspect that treatment centers using these ideas will be common some day in the future and will be much more successful than the standard treatment today, which all too often still consists of dumping alcoholics into hospitals and letting them dry out, with severe pain and suffering. When they are discharged, most go right back to the alcohol, the most dangerous and widely used street drug available without a prescription. The nutritional program outlined in this book may be the answer many people have been looking for.

A STILL UNSOLVED PROBLEM

As the Bible states, "The spirit is indeed willing, but the flesh is weak" (Matthew 26:41). One reason the body is weak is because of nutrient deficiencies. Another reason is because beverage alcohol is a slow-acting poison. Other alcohols are immediate poisons: if you add a carbon atom to drinking (ethyl) alcohol, you get C_3H_7OH (isopropyl or rubbing alcohol), which is toxic. CH_3OH (methanol) is found in windshield washer fluid and is just one carbon less than drinking alcohol . . . and again, is very toxic.

Alcohol abuse remains an unsolved problem, enormously costly and enormously painful. It is not just a problem of the young, either. Few people realize that over two-thirds of all hospital admissions of the elderly may be alcohol related.[1]

Alcohol use and abuse is common, and the problems it causes are enormous:

- Percentage of adults who drank alcohol in the year 2005: 61 percent.[2]

- Percentage of current drinkers who had five or more drinks on at least one day in the past year (data from 2005): 32 percent.[3]

- Number of annual alcohol-induced deaths, excluding accidents and homicides: 21,081.[4]

- Number of alcoholic liver disease deaths annually: 12,548.[5]

Beverage alcohol is a major factor in most violent crimes, notably sexual assault and murder. At least one-third, and some

TERMS OF ADDICTION

The word *addiction* has to work too hard. It is used to describe people who have such a passion for gambling that they will not let anything stand in the way of fulfilling this passion. It is used to describe people who cannot stop shopping. And, of course, it is used to describe people who cannot stop taking medication or street drugs even though they are being destroyed by this compulsive habit. We need different words to describe each of these obsessive-compulsive activities to which we humans are prone.

Voluntary Illegal—These activities are the best known: alcohol use past the point of impairment (but not the act of occasional drinking), and street drug addictions. The definition of precisely what is illegal varies from culture to culture, nation to nation, and even community to community. For example, there are still many dozens of "dry" counties and towns in the United States, where the sale of alcohol is against the law, regardless of age.

Social sanctions may grossly distort the clinical picture, since most drug addicts do not have enough means to provide for their addiction and livelihood. Such drugs include the hallucinogens, such as LSD, cocaine, and narcotics such as morphine and heroin. If they are going to maintain their addiction, addicts often see no choice but to turn to crime; they spend their addicted lives trying to get enough money to maintain the addiction.

Voluntary Legal—Perhaps the best example is methadone maintenance, a legally sanctioned addiction that allows the addict to obtain their drugs at a reasonable price so they can work and live. Some prefer this legal addiction, while others hate it just as much but know they have no alternative. Some drugs are always legal, such as the stimulant drug caffeine. Some drugs are sometimes legal, such as the prescription stimulant drugs Adderall, Ritalin, and Dexedrine. And some stimulant drugs are always illegal, such as crack cocaine. Age is a factor in legality.

One may wonder if a twenty-year-old is really all that much more irresponsible, and all that much more vulnerable to the effects of alcohol, than someone aged twenty-one.

Involuntary—This is a maladaptive pattern of substance use leading to clinically significant impairment or distress manifested by:

- Physical withdrawal symptoms

- Persistent or unsuccessful efforts to cut down or control substance use

- Important social, occupational, or recreational activities that are given up or reduced because of substance use

- Substance use that is continued despite knowledge of having persistent and recurrent physical or psychological problems caused or exacerbated by the substance

studies indicate as much as three-quarters, of all suicides are alcohol related. Alcohol directly kills about 40,000 drivers each year, not counting their passengers, pedestrians, and occupants of other cars. We have no love for the tobacco industry, which kills over 400,000 smokers annually. Still, smoking is unlikely to lead to murder over a piece of meatloaf, and alcohol literally has.[6] But like cigarettes, alcohol does lead to lung cancer, and cancers of the mouth, esophagus, larynx, tongue, throat, and much of the rest of the body.

Given all this and more, we are surely aware that alcohol is harmful to health. It causes malnutrition by displacing nourishing foods in the diet and by causing nutrient deficiencies, particularly the B vitamins. And it damages the liver and the brain.

Substance abuse continues despite knowledge of having persistent and recurrent physical or psychological problems caused or exacerbated by the substance. Depressive disorders often co-occur with anxiety disorders and substance abuse.[7] Drug-dependent people continue to use the drugs very often against their own will; it is no longer a voluntary choice for them. Some are willing to keep using them because they somehow expect that drugs will really help them recover, but when they are given another option—to go with a nutritional (orthomolecular) approach—they will do so with alacrity. Hardly anyone really likes to feel drugged. While this book is primarily about the orthomolecular treatment of alcoholics, it will also briefly address some nutritional methods to stop smoking and to prevent or moderate the withdrawal symptoms of caffeine and narcotic addictions.

A person whose drinking interferes with his or her psychological, social, and economic well-being is an alcoholic. This is not a derisory term but rather a description of the behavior that is occurring. It denotes no particular personality type, and it depends on a number of variables that make it individual. The amount consumed is not the major issue, although it is clear that the more one drinks, the more toxic are the effects. Some individuals are alcoholic even though they drink relatively small amounts of alcohol daily. One of my (A.H.) patients was admitted to the hospital suffering from delirium tremens (DTs), but when she recovered, I discovered that she drank only one cocktail each afternoon before dinner. Others, like former British prime minister Winston Churchill, consumed enormous amounts of alcohol, yet I don't think he was an alcoholic. Nor is the frequency of drinking helpful in determining who is an alcoholic. I treated a man who left home once every three months to have a weekend binge in another city; he remained abstinent until his next scheduled weekend binge.

Whether or not the alcohol is seriously interfering with a person's health depends on a number of factors. Food is the most important one. The effects of the alcohol are much less serious if one can also eat properly. Many alcoholics cannot afford to drink and eat well; if they eventually have to choose between eating and drinking, they may choose drinking as the more desirable option. Money is a main factor: if one can afford to live well and eat well, the pathological effect of the alcohol does not become evident so quickly. And finally, reputation and social situation are extremely important. A combination of Alcoholics Anonymous, social sanctions, and nutritional orthomolecular support can be very effective.

ORTHOMOLECULAR THERAPY FOR ALCOHOLISM

According to orthomolecular medicine, the basis for health is optimum nutrition. When malnutrition or nutrient starvation is present, it is impossible to respond effectively to any medical treatment. *Orthomolecular,* the word coined by Linus Pauling, Ph.D., in 1968, describes a method that uses nutrients and normal ("ortho") constituents of the body in optimum amounts as the main treatment. In his book *How to Live Longer and Feel Better,* Dr. Pauling wrote, "I believe that in general the treatment of disease by the use of substances such as ascorbic acid, that are normally present in the human body and are required for life, is to be preferred to treatment by the use of powerful synthetic substances or plant products, which may, and usually do, have undesirable side effects. Substances such as vitamin C and most of the other vitamins are remarkable for their low toxicity and absence of side effects when taken in amounts larger than those usually available in the diet. I have coined the term *orthomolecular medicine* for the preservation of good health and the treatment of disease by varying the concentration in the human body of substances that are normally present in the body and are required for health."[8] This definition has never been surpassed for its accuracy and its vision of the future for the treatment of disease.

Orthomolecular physicians use all modern treatments, including drugs, surgery, and physical and psychological methods, when these are appropriate. For example, when antidepressants or tranquilizers are needed, they are used in conjunction with the nutrients and nutritional recommendations. The drugs are used to gain rapid control over undesirable or disabling symptoms and are slowly withdrawn once the patient begins to respond to orthomolecular treatment. Since all people are healthier when they eat good food only (avoiding junk food), they can resist disease and injury more effectively when they are healthier due to optimum nutrition.

Orthomolecular nutrition, in contrast to "eat the food groups" nutrition, emphasizes the use of supplemental vitamins, minerals, and other accessory factors in amounts that are higher than those recommended by the government-sponsored "dietary allowances." Furthermore, orthomolecular nutrition is employed to treat illnesses that are not considered traditional deficiency diseases. Two examples would be using tens of thousands of milligrams of intravenous vitamin C to fight cancer or using several thousand milligrams of niacin per day to treat psychosis.

Orthomolecular physicians recognize that a large fraction of those with so-called psychiatric problems, including those suffering from depression and substance abuse issues, are ill due to physical factors. The usual tests do not reveal pathology. These physical factors are changes in metabolism and/or nutrition. When treated successfully, the psychiatric symptoms clear. Very little psychotherapy is required, and that can be given by any competent physician.

Alcoholism and drug addiction, so often portrayed as without cure, can indeed be ended with high-dose nutrient therapy. This may surprise many, anger a few, and, we hope, arouse your interest. Orthomolecular (megavitamin) therapy is cheaper, safer, and more effective than drugs or counseling. And the knowledge of this has been available for over fifty years.

Bill W. strongly advocated megavitamin therapy for alcoholism back in the 1950s and 1960s. Bill taught that there were three components to the treatment of alcoholism: spiritual, mental, and medical. Alcoholics Anonymous provided the spiritual home that alcoholics could not find anywhere else and helped them sustain abstinence. But for many, AA alone was not enough; not everyone in AA achieved a comfortable sobriety. Bill recognized that the other two components were important.

When he heard of our use of niacin for treating alcoholics, Bill became very enthusiastic about it because niacin gave these unfortunate patients immense relief from their chronic depression and other physical and mental complaints. I (A.H.) personally treated Bill for depression, using niacin. This vitamin regimen was so successful that Bill urged many others to try it. When they did, it worked for them too.

CHAPTER 2

WHAT CAUSES ADDICTIONS?

What causes addictions? There is no short answer to this question in spite of many decades of theorizing about it. None of the psychiatric hypotheses have been very helpful. Alcoholics Anonymous (AA) has been the most helpful, but even this very useful social program reaches only a small proportion of the total population, and only those who join AA are helped. AA is not based upon hypothesis—it is based on research in action, on actually seeing what works. Some of the causes of alcoholism are social, such as having alcohol freely available. Blaming the individual is not very useful, and we have not yet come across alcoholics who really enjoy their addicted state, yet they cannot free themselves from it.

One cause is the general nutritional deficiency of people who barely survive their modern, high-sugar, low-fiber, and very-low-vitamin diets. For example, the elderly characteristically eat poor diets, low in vitamins, low in protein, low in fiber . . . and remarkably *high* in alcohol. Quiet drinkers they may be, but the problem is serious and widespread. An incredible two-thirds of all hospital admissions of the elderly may be alcohol-related.[1]

We are all naturally inclined to avoid, and to seek relief from, pain and discomfort. Sometimes we will use anything that will achieve this. Bill W., cofounder of AA, described the evening he became alcoholic. He was at a party and not enjoying it one bit and he wondered why the other people were having so much fun. He was persuaded to have one drink, and suddenly his world opened and he understood the drawing power of alcohol.

We are convinced that healthy people will not become alcoholics. They will drink, if they do, in moderation. Only people who are not healthy become alcoholics. The undernourished body accepts alcohol gratefully until the person becomes addicted, then it is not so grateful. We would go so far as to state it as a law: *only the sick become alcoholic.*

When alcoholics can afford to both eat and drink, especially if their food is more nutritious than the usual American diet, they will suffer less from nutrient deficiencies. However, too many cannot afford both and will prefer the alcohol, which gives them calories free of any useful nutrients. This will make their alcoholism more severe and more progressive.

PATIENT OR BOOZE HOUND: WHAT'S IN A NAME?

When I (A.W.S.) asked my college students to state specific symptomatic and behavioral differences between "heavy drinking" and "alcoholism," they had trouble doing it. That is not a total surprise. I know many alcoholics, and I know many heavy drinkers. You probably do too. So, which is which? Is a person who drinks six or more martinis a day an alcoholic? Is a person who drinks a six-pack or more of beer per day just a heavy drinker? The amount of alcohol in six beers is virtually the same as six martinis. I used to invite my students to consider the definition of "binge drinker": five drinks in a row. Few students wanted to characterize themselves as "binge drinkers" even though many, by definition, were. What is the essential difference, then, if you are a binge drinker downing a six-pack four or five days a week or an alcoholic drinking seven or eight shots of bourbon five or six days a week? Is it just a matter of one or two more drinks per day, or two more days per week, that makes you an alcoholic?

Generally, it is said that a heavy drinker can stop and an alcoholic can't. Yet the behavior (number of drinks a day) is very similar. Generally, it is said that an alcoholic has a life seriously impaired by drinking. Tell that to a police officer who pulls over a binge-drinking driver who is DUI (driving under the influence). The officer will not ask Dorothy's proverbial question, "Are you a good witch or a bad witch?" The officer will measure the alcohol, note the impairment, and run the offender in. When I was a young man, the fellow who shared my office was fired for drinking on the job. He was not an alcoholic, but it didn't matter. His life was seriously impaired by his drinking. Thus, the definitions blur.

Children of alcoholics are much more likely to become alcoholic than other children. Still, the majority of these children do *not* become alcoholic. Certainly, genetics influences alcoholism—after all, genes influence pretty much everything—but if there is a sure-to-cause-alcoholism gene, science has yet to find it.

One clear advantage of the label "alcoholic" is that it provides a medical diagnosis that enables the alcoholic to receive medical care covered by insurance. A "heavy drinker" may not get the same assistance. One reason for this is that the "heavy drinker" is often seen as choosing a bad behavior, whereas the alcoholic is seen as a sick person who simply cannot help it.

We think the emphasis on "sick" should be changed to an emphasis on "nutrient deprived." Our view is not the view of AA, although we wish to emphasize that we strongly support AA's mission and are convinced that AA has helped many people. We think, as did Bill W., that far more people would be helped if they had large doses of niacin, vitamin C, and the rest of the orthomolecular nutrient program presented in this book. *It does not matter how the drinking started or what name you want to give it. The bottom line is this: high doses of nutrients stop excessive drinking.*

SUGAR: THE FIRST ADDICTION

We believe that addictions begin during infancy. One suspicious factor starts very early: baby formulas are commonly made up of cow's milk and sugar. This may be the basis of a food addiction later in life, especially among bottle-fed infants, to one of their main foods: cow's milk. Sugar is the first major addicting substance, and many children are just as addicted to sugar as alcoholics are to alcohol. Alcohol, a very simple carbohydrate, is similar to sugar. We know of one boy, seven years old, who was seen crawling on his hands and knees to the kitchen in the middle of the night to reach the sugar bowl, and he gulped down the sugar by the handful. The sweet taste, so essential to animals in deciding which foods are ripe and safe, becomes one of the main factors in creating the addiction. Later, many of these children as teenagers are addicted to milk. In some cases, they drink huge amounts each day, as much as half of their calories. But as they grow older and have access to alcohol, many find that this makes them feel better than either sugar or milk could, and they become addicted to alcohol. At Alcoholics Anonymous meetings, members often drink coffee super-saturated with sugar.

And let's not forget that children commonly drink colas laced with caffeine on top of high sugar content: twelve or more teaspoons of sugar in a single can of soda. According to the Center for Science in the Public Interest, "Soda pop is Americans' single biggest source of refined sugars. . . . Twelve- to nineteen-year-old boys get 44 percent of their thirty-four teaspoons of sugar a day from soft drinks. Girls get 40 percent of their twenty-four teaspoons of sugar from soda. Because some people drink little soda pop, the percentages are higher among actual drinkers."[2]

The crossover between a sugarholic and an alcoholic is illustrated by this patient's letter:

> All my forty-five-plus years, I've fought against sugar,
> refined carbohydrates, and the fatigue and mood swings

they bring about. However, like an alcoholic, I always seem to end up craving, and then getting back with sugar products.

I read the following post on an Internet newsgroup: "In order to control your addiction, follow the protocol for alcohol at www.doctoryourself.com/alcohol_protocol. html. My daughter treated a sugar addiction nutritionally exactly as alcoholism is treated, and it works. Many people who have sugar addiction have alcoholics in the family. When alcoholics go off alcohol, they nearly always start eating lots of sugar. Unfortunately, this usually keeps the addiction going."

I'd love to see a diet and tactics developed to get off a sugar addiction. I am the son of alcoholics, and I'm addicted to a terrible sugar and refined carbohydrate diet that leaves me exhausted and stressed out. Your assertion that alcoholism can be "cured" really is heresy to my way of thinking, but maybe you might be right. I would like to find a nutritional key that might help me in my ongoing white-knuckled struggle as I hurry past the baked goods and candy.

Probably the most reliable and most powerful help for the sugar junkie is indeed to diligently follow the nutritional program for alcoholism developed by Roger J. Williams, Ph.D., author of *Alcoholism: The Nutritional Approach* (Austin, TX: University of Texas Press, 1959). Large quantities of the B-complex vitamins are a cornerstone of the treatment. We think that the cheap and easy key is to take the entire B-complex at least six times daily. Chromium, vitamin C, lecithin, the amino acid L-glutamine, and a vegetable-rich, high-fiber, complex-carbohydrate diet are also very important. See Chapter 4 for details of our nutritional program.

THE CONNECTION TO ADDICTIVE FOODS

The idea that foods are addictive is not generally accepted in medicine. Orthomolecular physicians, who understand this connection, have no problem with it. Over the past forty years, I (A.H.) have been surprised at the number of patients who were depressed and who also had a history of many different types of allergic reactions, such as asthma, hay fever, rashes, frequent colds, and sinus problems. For a long time, I accepted this and did not see any connection until I became aware that the biochemical problems causing the allergic reactions were also causing the depression.

Since then, I have treated hundreds of depressed men and women who had not responded to medication. They became well when the food causing the allergy was identified and removed from their diets. In almost every case, patients were able to discover what food they were allergic to—it could be any food, but usually it was one of the staples, such as milk, sugar, wheat, or eggs. When patients started an elimination diet, they might go through a "withdrawal," which can be mild or very severe, almost as if they had suddenly stopped taking heroin. One of my patients became severely depressed and suicidal on the second day of her diet without dairy products. I had to admit her to a hospital, and we watched her while she continued the diet; five days later she was normal. Milk products were the cause of her depression.

I advise patients to expect a week of withdrawal. The allergic foods are identified by a nutritional history, and the diagnosis is confirmed by an elimination diet followed by a challenge test. But if more than one food is suspected, they may have to first do a four- or five-day water fast.

Alcoholics may be unusually allergic to the very grains or fruits that are used to make the alcohol. One patient of mine was admitted with delirium tremens (DTs), violent tremors caused by withdrawal from alcohol. He was watched, given lots of water, and was well in a few days. When he was later given potatoes, he had a grand mal convulsion. When he was given wheat, he became as befuddled as if he had had a drink of alcohol.

We suspect that food allergies act primarily on the gastrointestinal system and interfere with its functions in the following ways. Allergy may increase peristalsis and cause diarrhea, sometimes severe. Crohn's disease may be one of these gluten allergic diseases. It may also make the gut more permeable to larger polypeptide fragments, which penetrate more easily into the blood and flash into the brain in seconds. And it interferes with the availability of some nutrients. Some babies suffer from milk-induced iron deficiency, and we have seen many who have the signs of zinc deficiency (white areas on their nails, stretch marks, pale complexion, and growing pains in childhood). If these factors are all operative, the long-term use of these foods will lead to serious deficiencies in vitamins and minerals. People with one or more food allergies can be placed on a comprehensive, multinutrient supplementation program.

The great biochemist Roger J. Williams, Ph.D., taught two key points: biochemical individuality and genetotrophics. These five-dollar words simply mean that:

1. We are all different.

2. The genes express themselves in relation to nutrients available to the body.

Food allergies are one confounding factor in a complex, unique-to-you human body made up of trillions of cells undergoing thousands of chemical reactions. Everybody is different, and food allergies vary from person to person. That is why we have personal physicians.

In general, we think food allergies can aggravate or cause many illnesses, probably by aggravating the great underlying cause: malnutrition. We are convinced that poor nutrition can predispose to alcohol abuse and drug abuse. In addition to eliminating the trouble-makers in our diet, we also need to eat more of the good things. Getting rid of sugar and food additives is a you-can't-miss proposition. You will not die if you avoid milk products; most mammals do not drink any milk at all after weaning. You will not die of artificial chemical food additive deficiency. Nor will you die from a lack of processed sugar. And you will most certainly not die from taking vitamin supplements and eating a wholesome diet! Many suffer from eating poorly—no one dies from eating right.

CHAPTER 3

NIACIN FOR ALCOHOLISM: HOW IT ALL BEGAN

In 1950, I (A.H.) started my new career in psychiatry. I had completed my rotating internship at City Hospital in Saskatoon, Canada, had gotten my doctorate in agricultural biochemistry at the University of Minnesota, had done research developing methods for analyzing vitamins in cereal and flour products, and had become interested in psychiatry. To my surprise, the director of psychiatric services in the Department of Public Health in Saskatchewan accepted my proposal that I start a research program in psychiatry.

I had the advantage that I knew no psychiatry and was therefore not loaded up with the usual stuff that medical students have to put up with. I was also appointed consultant to the pathologist at the General Hospital in Regina. The Munro Wing was a small psychiatric building separate from the rest of the hospital with thirty-eight beds on two wards. It was the only psychiatric ward in a general hospital in the province of Saskatchewan and accepted every type of psychiatric disorder, including alcoholics who were suffering from delirium tremens (DTs). I had time to learn something about psychiatry in seminars, conferences, individual instruction, and in many vigorous case discussions. Our patients came to us in rotation, and since there were four residents, I received every fourth admission.

A few alcoholics suffering from DTs were admitted. There was no specific treatment for these unfortunate patients and the mortality rate was as high as 20 percent of all their admissions. Dr. Jonathan Gould, a psychiatrist in England, had reported that large doses of the B-complex vitamins and glucose were very effective in treating delirious states, including acute alcoholic psychosis.[1] The two major vitamins were ascorbic acid (vitamin C) and thiamine (B_1), with smaller amounts of niacinamide (B_3) and pyridoxine (B_6).

With my colleague Dr. Humphry Osmond, I developed a treatment protocol for alcoholics in DTs or in a predeleriod state. On admission, they were given niacin (500 milligrams I.V. and 3 grams oral) and ascorbic acid (2,000 mg). On the first day, they received niacin (3,000 mg) after each of three meals, the same amount of vitamin C, and a sedative, if needed. This was to be continued until they were free of the delirium. The results were very dramatic. When used as recommended, most cases of delirium tremens and acute alcoholic intoxications respond well within twenty-four hours. For this, it is as good as the tranquilizers commonly used at the time, but it has the added advantage that there is no sedation. The patient remains more alert and, after a few hours, is cooperative. There are no toxic complications. Our studies in Saskatchewan corroborated Dr. Gould's observations in England. These doses were much larger than the usual recommended daily doses.

We started to use these higher doses for the treatment of schizophrenia, with no toxicity and with major effectiveness. We did not specifically treat alcoholics in our double-blind, controlled trials of niacin. As I began to enlarge the number of patients on vitamin B_3, it soon became clear that many schizophrenic patients were also alcoholic. The dual diagnosis classification was not then considered a major problem; it occurred in about 10 percent of my schizophrenic patients. With vitamin B_3 therapy, both conditions were much improved. Soon, I was using niacin for alcoholics who were not drinking, who were members of AA, and who still suffered from marked anxiety and depression.

Some schizophrenic patients drank alcohol as a self-treatment, because they preferred to be drunk rather than suffer hallucinations. In one case from 1960, a young woman suffered from both problems. She had discovered that whenever she joined AA and remained abstinent for several weeks, her voices (which had been terrible) returned and she would start drinking again. She was faced with this dreadful choice: to be drunk and free of hallucinations, or to be sober and suffer the hallucinations. She came to me for help. I offered her a third way, and after she started taking niacin, she recovered from both. Later, she became one of the original members of Schizophrenics Anonymous, which started in Saskatoon in 1960.

VITAMIN B$_3$: BILL W.'S FAVORITE VITAMIN

I met Bill W. (William Griffith Wilson), cofounder of Alcoholics Anonymous (AA), at a meeting in New York in 1958. After that, Bill and I became close friends. I introduced him to vitamin B$_3$ (niacin) and suggested that he try it. He had been suffering from severe tension, fatigue, and insomnia for many years, although he did not let that deter him from his important work at the AA International Headquarters. A few weeks after he started taking niacin (1,000 mg after each of three meals for a total of 3 grams a day), his fatigue, chronic tension, insomnia, and discomfort disappeared.

Bill immediately became a strong supporter of our work with niacin, but he did not leave it at that. He told his colleagues and friends about his own recovery and discussed the research we were doing in Saskatchewan. He was aware of the extraordinary properties of vitamin B$_3$ from his discussions with me and his examination of the medical literature.

Bill was not shy about passing on this information, much to the chagrin of the International Board of AA. He had created this board and, many years before, had invited physicians to become members. They were all friends of his, but the doctors on the board were not happy with Bill and accused him of meddling with medical matters, which were none of his business. Bill did not agree—his business was to help as many alcoholics as possible get well, and if vitamins were going to help, he was all in favor of using them. And he knew that vitamins were extraordinarily safe. But this was news to the doctors, who were not aware that vitamins in large or optimum doses had properties they did not have when used in the very low, usual doses then being recommended.

I remember two examples Bill told me about. One was a man with severe arthritis, who found it very difficult to continue his job as a gardener. Bill told him about niacin, and after he was on this vitamin for a while, his arthritis vanished. This was another confirmation of Dr. William Kaufman's excellent research between 1940 and 1950. By 1949, Dr. Kaufman had published two books summarizing his studies on arthritis, *The Common Form of Niacinamide Deficiency Disease: Aniacinamidosis* and *The Common Form of Joint Dysfunction, Its Incidence and Treatment.*[2] These were very careful, clinically controlled experiments on many hundreds of arthritics, in which he showed that most of the patients given the vitamin became normal, or so much better they were no longer seriously handicapped.

Another example from Bill was a wealthy individual from the West Coast who called him up very depressed. He had been suffering from manic-depressive (now called bipolar) disease for many years and had been helped somewhat by a psychoanalyst. However, his psychoanalyst died and he had become severely depressed. Bill told him that he would send him a jug of niacin (500 mg tablets) and that he should take two tablets (1,000 mg) three times daily. Within a few months, his friend was without the need of any more psychiatric treatment. The more people Bill told about niacin, and the more responses he saw, the more convinced he was of the merit in our work.

Bill went even further. One evening when I was visiting him at his downtown hotel in New York, he pulled out thirty files and said, "Abram, I want to show you the results of my research." He had given niacin to thirty of his associates and friends in AA after carefully telling them about niacin and its properties, how much to take, and so on. After one month, ten of them were well. After two months, another ten were well. And after three months, the last ten had not responded. I was delighted and impressed, as his response rate was very similar to what I was seeing in my practice. Bill W. was thus the first layperson to repeat our research trials and to confirm our findings, but of course his study was not done according to the clinical "gold standard" of the double-blind test.

Seeking Support for Niacin

Bill realized that the use of a vitamin for alcoholism needed medical support. In 1966, he was invited by the International Doctors in Alcoholics Anonymous to address their annual convention in Indianapolis, Indiana. For some time before that, Bill had been reluctant to continue his previous policy of speaking frequently at AA meetings and conventions as he did not want to be deified. He had previously refused to accept invitations from this medical group. This time, he asked me if I would also come and talk to these doctors, and I agreed. Bill told them that he would come and speak to them, but only if they also invited me. They were delighted to invite me (they would have invited the devil if only it brought Bill along).

At the convention, I was surrounded by a large number of doctors who had never heard of me but who surely were delighted that Bill was there. It was soon obvious that these AA doctors knew very little about nutrition and about the pernicious effect of sugar on their health. One doctor arrived with a large box of chocolate bars and I was told that he did this every year—he would hand out bars freely to anyone who suffered from excessive anxiety and tension! "Dry drunks" were common among alcoholics, even if they had been not been drinking. Often, they would be so tense that one would suspect they had been drinking.

I had been an observer at a few AA meetings and had seen that the most popular drink was coffee with enough sugar left at the bottom of the cup that it amounted to drinking saturated sucrose solutions with a lot of caffeine. By then, I had given several hundred alcoholics a glucose tolerance test and had found that all of them suffered from hypoglycemia. This term was very unpopular as doctors thought that only "quacks" would use the term *hypoglycemia*. Now it is called type 2 diabetes, and there seems to be no opposition to that term. A "dry drunk" was a person whose blood sugar was so low that they could not function properly, and of course a chocolate bar would elevate the sugar and bring them out of that reaction. But that is not the correct continuing treatment, as using sugar simply aggravates the condition.

Bill was a very charismatic and clear speaker, and he enthralled the doctors with his stories of what niacin had done for him and for many of his friends. Then I spoke about the work we were doing in Canada. At the end of that morning session, the meeting appointed a committee of three doctors to examine our claims.

Today, if any other group had appointed a committee to examine this question, it would never be completed. First, the committee would have to write up a very comprehensive grant proposal, which would be submitted to some granting body, a government agency, or research institute. But it would have to be cleared by a research review committee and by the ethics committee. Research today is so complicated and so full of red tape, which serves no useful purpose, that it often becomes a chore and never gets done. We were not hindered this way many years ago. The committee appointed at the meeting acted quickly. All three took niacin themselves and after a month felt so much better that they approved it. No grants, no fuss, and no bother. The three members became pioneers in the use of niacin for treating alcoholics and schizophrenic patients and began to spread the information to members of the association. Of course, vitamins are safe and the essential safeguards involving testing drugs are not necessary.

Unfortunately, physicians knowing very little about vitamins consider them nearly as toxic as drugs.

The psychiatric establishment on the East Coast heard about Bill's interest and became very concerned. It selected a young psychiatrist to write a rebuttal to my message, even though he had not been at the meeting. This rebuttal was circulated and a copy sent to Bill, who promptly sent it to me. I was astonished by the poor quality of that document, which was full of errors of fact, was badly written, and had little relevance to what Bill and I had discussed at that meeting. That young psychiatrist eventually rose to a high rank in U.S. psychiatry.

CHAPTER 4

CONQUERING ALCOHOLISM NUTRITIONALLY

Alcohol consumption and abuse is more widespread and more serious than most persons imagine. Two-thirds of all American adults drink alcohol, averaging about three drinks per day, seven days a week, fifty-two weeks a year. If you do not drink that much, then somebody out there is drinking more. Those are the heavy drinkers, as numerous as one adult in ten.

We need to collectively and individually stop or greatly reduce our use of alcohol. A general ban on alcohol has already been tried. Prohibition (from 1920 to 1933 in the United States) is usually written off as a failed social experiment, but the truth is that alcohol-related hospital admissions and deaths did indeed decline during Prohibition's early years. Individual action requires no law. Many alcoholics have stopped using alcohol by willpower alone. If you are in Alcoholics Anonymous (AA), abstinence is supported by the help of the power of a Will greater than your own. If it works, do it.

More alcohol users and abusers could "work the steps" of AA, or just plain stop drinking on their own, if they were optimally nourished. If you drink too much, then you are not eating right. Malnourished alcoholics consume significantly more ethanol. The specific vitamin deficiencies present in a substantial proportion of the population are directly related to alcohol consumption.[1]

- Alcohol is filling, so it displaces more nourishing foods in the diet, which causes malnutrition.[2]

- Alcohol causes thiamine (vitamin B_1) deficiency in particular and a deficiency of many other nutrients as well. Alcoholics frequently have evidence of malnutrition because of decreased intake and impaired absorption of nutrients.[3]

- Alcohol destroys the liver and brain, gradually but profoundly. This damage *increases* the need for nutrients to repair these organs at a time when the drinker is eating fewer and fewer good foods.[4] For instance, chronic alcohol-related brain damage can often be a direct result of nutrient depletion, particularly thiamine, vitamin B_{12}, nicotinamide, and B_6.[5]

Thus, a healthy diet is the first critical step. Vitamins and other food supplements are also essential for the heavy drinker. Roger J. Williams, Ph.D., and many others have been advocating this nutritional approach for over half a century.

START WITH A HEALTHY DIET

Nutrition is the key. The quality of the diet must be improved, and the easiest way is to use a no-junk diet. We define "junk" as any food to which sugar has been added. If these foods are excluded, this will also remove about 90 percent of other junk chemicals that are routinely added to our processed foods. This definition also includes refined flour of any type. It is a stiff definition. The only way to appreciate it is to try it.

In addition, many patients are mentally sick because they are allergic to one or more foods, usually staples—the common foods are milk and any products derived from it, wheat, coffee or tea, chocolate, and more. These can often be identified by the dietary history. If a food is suspected, it is eliminated from the diet for one month. If at the end of that trial the patient is much better, the same food is reintroduced in a so-called challenge test. It will bring back the same symptoms from which the patient had been suffering. But sometimes it is impossible to determine what the offending foods are so a four-day or five-day water fast may be needed, followed by the reintroduction of foods (one food at each meal).

I (A.H.) have treated hundreds of patients who recovered when the offending foods were removed. A young man, age twenty-two, complained that he had been depressed all his life. On the dairy elimination diet, he was well in two weeks. He then did the challenge test by eating some ice cream, and two hours later he was very depressed again; one hour after that, he was agitated and almost psychotic. The police were called in to restrain him. He fell asleep for three hours in the morning and has been well since.

Indeed, lime sherbet makes me (A.W.S.) crazy. That is not a figure of speech, merely implying that I'd really like to eat it. Rather, it means that eating it literally makes me "nuts." I still vividly recall, as a young man, having a double-scoop cone of the chartreuse-green stuff. About thirty minutes later, I was, to use my grandmother's expression, fit to be tied: agitated, irritable, and angry. I could barely control my behavior and certainly could not control how I felt. When the haze cleared, I wondered what the heck had happened.

It finally dawned on me that it might be my reaction to the load of sugar and artificial color that I had just ingested. As Dr. Lendon H. Smith has said, if you crave a food, it is probably bad for you. To this day, I am cautious about consuming sugar, and I do not eat artificially colored foods of any kind.

It isn't just me, and it isn't just anecdotal. Long dismissed by medical authorities, sugar, food colorings, and other all-too-common food additives do indeed adversely affect mood. In a study involving 277 preschool children, conducted by the Southampton General Hospital in England, artificial food colorings and other additives increased hyperactive behavior. Researchers stated that "children's hyperactivity fell after withdrawal of food additives from the children's diets (and) there was an increase in hyperactivity when food additives were reintroduced."[6] If you have ever been around kids on the day after Halloween, you already know this.

A Toxic Pseudo-Food

The most toxic, the most attractive, and the most addicting pseudo-food is sugar. There are several kinds of dietary sugars. The primary one is sucrose or table sugar, a disaccharide (two-ring sugar) made from one molecule each of glucose and fructose. It is digested by splitting the molecule and releasing each of the single-ring (monosaccharide) sugars.

Glucose is the sugar that is most important to the body. This does not mean that one needs to go out of one's way to eat it, as all your dietary carbohydrates are broken down into glucose, which is then absorbed and metabolized. Glucose is the least toxic of the sugars.

Fructose is more troublesome, as it is harder for the body to metabolize and use properly. As the name suggests, it is present in fruit. But much more is consumed through processed foods containing corn syrup, which is high in fructose. With the advent of high-tech foods, this monosaccharide has become a major part of our total sugar intake. We think it should be avoided even more assiduously than glucose and sucrose. Foods rich in fructose should be eaten in very small amounts. Soft drinks, candy, and highly processed foods are the worst.

The least common sugar is lactose, which is found in milk. Like sucrose, it is a disaccharide, made from glucose and galactose. Many children lose the enzyme that splits this sugar as they mature, and they become intolerant of lactose.

None of the sugars are really "foods." Rather, they are purpose-specific chemical extracts from plant foods, and (aside from calories) have zero nutrition. The plants from which they are made have lots of nutrients; the processed extracts have none. In case we have not made our position clear enough—sugars are junk. *The degree of unhealthiness of a food is determined by the amount of sugars that are present in that food.* It is just that simple. Yes, fats and processed carbohydrates are no boon to health, either. A modern doughnut—made from white flour, soaked and cooked in oil, and full of sugar both inside and outside—is the perfect example of what is wrong with modern diets.

Simple Nutritional Rules

Simply put, alcoholics should avoid all foods they are allergic to. *If you crave it, it is probably bad for you.* A good plant-based diet and plenty of fresh vegetable juices are important. A mostly vegetarian diet effortlessly ensures better health. More fiber and complex carbohydrates; less fat and sugar. No junk food! We keep saying it, because it is so very important.

A cross-over, double-blind study was made of twenty alcoholics to see if dietary corrections changed their subjective symptoms. In one group, the diet was corrected to meet all the Recommended Dietary Allowances (RDAs) of nutrients; a control group of alcoholics was given a placebo. After ninety days, subjects in the first group subjectively reported having more energy, less confusion, and felt "mellow." Psychological tests showed improvement, vitamin levels improved, and the nutritional analysis was normal. The second group had essentially no improvement. The groups were then switched for ninety days, with similar results. "When all the alcoholic groups were placed on the supplement and dietary regime, the psychologist and alcohol counselors reported the group's therapy was more productive and proceeded at a faster rate than those on the normal halfway house diets," reported C. Jean Poulos, Sc.D., Ph.D. "Apparently alcoholics are sufficiently depleted nutritionally that bringing the nutrients to RDA levels results in both subjective and objective changes."[7]

Controlled vegetable juice fasting has also been successfully used to clear out fatty livers. Juice fasting, along with large amounts of the B vitamins and vitamin C, may be a real long-term help for cirrhosis of the liver. The liver can regenerate to a considerable extent. Max Gerson, M.D., developer of the famous diet therapy for cancer and other diseases, said that it takes about eighteen months to do so. It is no surprise, then, that the Gerson Therapy focuses on the liver and on raw vegetable juice therapy.[8]

VITAMINS AND OTHER SUPPLEMENTS

There is no magic formula that works for everyone; as with shoes, one size does not fit all. Any combination of a large number of nutrients may be needed. The decision will be made based on the experience of the therapist and on existing laboratory tests. Vitamin B_3, especially the niacin form, should almost always be one of the main therapeutic nutrients.

A high-potency daily multivitamin/multimineral supplement is a good place to start. It should contain carotene (10,000–30,000 IU), an antioxidant and especially safe form of vitamin A. Additional vitamin E (400–800 IU) and selenium (50 mcg) should also be taken.

Vitamin B_3 (Niacin)

Take niacin (several hundred to several thousand milligrams per day), along with the rest of the B-complex vitamins (50 mg, six times daily). Excess consumption of either sugar or alcohol is known to increase the need for the vitamins necessary for their metabolism, specifically the B-complex vitamins. It is safest, easiest, and cheapest to take the whole B-vitamin team together.

The B vitamins, including much-needed niacin and thiamine, help correct a bad diet and also help level out low blood sugar problems. Hypoglycemia is often a factor in alcohol cravings. The body wants simple, quick carbohydrates, and we erroneously satisfy that craving with sugar or booze. Additionally, niacin helps the body to calm down. The B vitamins have been successfully used for decades by orthomolecular psychiatrists to relieve depression and psychoses, and they can also relieve the delirium tremens (DTs). Incidentally, you can create the symptoms of delirium tremens in laboratory animals without alcohol just by inducing B-vitamin deficiency.

There are two main forms of B_3: niacin and nicotinamide (or niacinamide). The term *vitamin B_3* refers to these two forms and to the nicotinamide adenine dinucleotide system, NAD and NADH (NADH is the reduced form and more active than NAD). Vitamin B_3 deficiency means a deficiency of niacin or niacinamide, or of NAD or NADH. Bill W. restored the designation "vitamin B_3" to the medical literature: in preparing his communications to AA physicians, he felt that vitamin B_3 would be much more appealing than the chemical names. He was right. The designation gradually came back into the medical literature and is now recognized worldwide.

Russell F. Smith, M.D., reported a trial of high-dose niacin in 500 diagnosed alcoholics over five years. Ten percent of the sample group were physically and emotionally intact, early intervention alcoholics; 40 percent were alcoholics with advanced physical symptoms; the final group were classical "low-bottom" alcoholics with serious physical and personal complications. Niacin showed potential for benefiting the alcoholic, particularly those demonstrating more serious central nervous system symptoms of the disease.

- Niacin improved sleep patterns, mood stability, and overall functioning in 60 percent of the test group who showed the more serious organic symptoms.

- Niacin significantly reduced acquired tolerance to alcohol.

- Niacin appeared to significantly shorten the course of the acute toxic brain syndrome.

- Niacin all but eliminated "dry drunk syndrome," including hyperexcitable, manic episodes, and suicidal depressions.

One theoretical basis for this activity appears to lie in the metabolism of 5-OH-tryptamine, or the monoamine oxidase (MAO) reaction. The breakdown of 5-OH-tryptamine into serotonin, dopamine, noradrenaline, and niacin may explain the phenomena in the clinical trial. These psychoactive substances are responsible for sensory perception, sleep, appetite, mood, and alertness. Levels are partially regulated through controlled degradation to inactive metabolites through the MAO reaction. Niacin could be a biochemical governor regulating the levels of these catecholamines.[9]

Another possible explanation involves acetaldehyde. Alcohol is metabolized in the body in two stages. First, it is metabolized by enzymes (alcohol dehydrogenase and aldehyde dehydrogenase) that require NAD as a coenzyme. In alcoholics, this stage reaction is faster than normal. Second, the metabolism of acetaldehyde to acetate is decreased in alcoholics. The result is an accumulation of acetaldehyde in the blood and the brain. Acetaldehyde then combines with dopamine to form morphine-like compounds that lead to addiction. The likely mechanism of action for niacin treatment is that niacin reduces acetaldehyde levels in the brain.[10]

The usual starting dose of niacin is 500–1,000 mg, taken immediately after meals, three times daily. But if one is worried about the intensity of the flush, one can start with 100 mg and increase it slowly. Niacin is much better tolerated when given with vitamin C. Gram-sized doses of vitamin C enhance a person's niacin tolerance; take at least as much vitamin C per dose as niacin. To repeat: vitamin B_3 must be given at least three times daily. It is water-soluble and very quickly excreted. This makes it very safe, as the levels cannot build up, but it also means B_3 has to be taken frequently and regularly to be effective.

The dose of niacin seldom needs to go above 2 grams taken

three times daily (6,000 mg per day total). It may be increased, but eventually the patient will develop nausea and later vomiting if the dose is too high. Each person is different. The optimum dose range is very wide. The same doses are used with niacinamide, but the optimum dose range is narrower, as more people develop nausea with niacinamide above 6 grams daily. Children are more tolerant to these doses. The dose is not related to size, age, or body weight. Some children will not complain of nausea; rather, they lose their appetite. The dose needs to be intelligently adjusted to get maximum benefits.

Potential Niacin Side Effects

Niacin has been used in doses up to tens of thousands of milligrams per day for over forty years by psychiatrists.[11] It is an effective alternative treatment for severe depression, psychotic behavior, and schizophrenia, as well as alcohol addiction.

Niacin is also one of the team of B-complex vitamins and any massive intake needs to be at least partly balanced with the rest of the B vitamins. Taking only one B vitamin is neither logical nor efficient, so avoid doing it unless there is a good reason.

In some patients, niacin will increase liver function tests, which does not always mean underlying liver pathology. Many other medicines cause the same elevations of liver function tests. Usually after a few days, the test results become normal whether or not niacin is still being taken. But to prevent confusing liver damage with increased activity, it is best to stop the niacin for five days and then do the tests. Working hard, the human liver can detoxify about one drink every two hours. Know anyone who drinks at a faster rate than that? Then marvel that they have a liver that functions at all. The liver undergoes profound changes in both its endoplasmic reticula and its microsomal enzymes in order to detoxify alcohol. The liver needs a chance to detoxify itself after it has detoxified your body. An overloaded liver may be temporarily overtaxed in an alcohol-strained system. This may be where some changes in liver function tests come from.[12]

A recent review of niacin finds that "the side effects of niacin have limited its use in general clinical practice. . . . Overall, the perception of niacin side effects is often greater than the reality."[13] There are a few niacin side effects that may be a nuisance but are not toxic reactions. Apart from a very few people who are allergic to the pills, most of these reactions are dose related. Patients must be informed of the possible side effects, both positive and negative.

Niacin usually causes a flush a few minutes after it is taken. The "niacin flush" begins in the forehead and works its way down the body, although only rarely affecting the toes. The higher the initial dose, the greater is the initial flush; however, if any dose causes a maximum flush, a larger dose taken later will not cause any greater flush. The capillaries are dilated and the blood flow through the organs is increased. This internal increase in blood flow, as well as in the skin, may last up to several hours. You should be aware that this will happen, otherwise you may be very surprised and even shocked. Consider starting on lower doses until you have adjusted to the decreased intensity of the flush, then the doses may be increased gradually.

Each time the niacin is taken, the flush is repeated but to a much lesser degree. In most cases, after a week or so, it is almost completely gone and is a minor nuisance at worst. If the routine is interrupted for several days and then resumed, the same sequence of flushing will occur, but the initial flush will usually not be as strong as the original one. The intensity of the flush is minimized by taking the pills after meals and by taking them regularly, in divided doses, three times daily. However, some people do not tolerate the flush and will have to discontinue taking niacin.

The good news is that nonflush niacin preparations are available. Niacinamide generally does not cause flushing except in a small percentage of people in whom it will cause an unpleasant flush (they probably convert the niacinamide too rapidly into niacin); for these people, it cannot be used. Very high doses of niacinamide can cause nausea. Inositol hexaniacinate is a nonflush niacin that virtually all sensitive persons can use. Even in high doses, it almost never causes nausea. Inositol hexaniacinate usually costs more than niacinamide.

Most patients will tolerate niacin if it is put to them in a positive way, but physicians who downplay its positive properties and overemphasize its potential problems will find that most patients will not remain on it. Orthomolecular physicians find a very high compliance rate.

Vitamin B$_6$ (Pyridoxine)

Alcohol users in general, and alcoholics in particular, typically have low or very low blood levels of vitamin B$_6$.[14] Kryptopyrole (also known as the "mauve factor") is found in the urine of some alcoholics. While it is not a specific cause of excessive drinking, its presence increases the likelihood one will use alcohol to relieve anxiety. Although the relationship between pyridoxine and alcohol is not as clear-cut as is the connection between niacin and alcoholism, there is ample evidence to recommend extra vitamin B$_6$ for persons who consume alcohol, and for those who are trying to stop consuming it.[15]

The usual dose range is 100–1,000 mg daily. Early in the development of orthomolecular psychiatry, the pioneer physicians freely used up to 3,000 mg daily and did not see any complications. The main indication is for those patients who excrete too much kryptopyrole in their urine. Both pyridoxine and the mineral zinc are used when this factor is present in excess.

Potential Pyridoxine Side Effects

Vitamin B$_6$ has been reported to cause temporary neurological symptoms, such as heaviness, tingling, or numbness of the limbs, in persons taking very large doses. It is very important to realize that such cases are not common, and when they do occur they usually result from huge doses of pyridoxine taken alone. The B vitamins are a team, and work best as a team. Upsetting the bal-

MEGAVITAMIN THERAPY FOR ANXIETY AND DEPRESSION

Vitamin therapy is effective for reducing levels of anxiety and depression among alcoholics. Individuals who are alcoholics are prone to experience elevated levels of anxiety and depression, and they also tend to use alcohol to self-medicate for relief. Researchers examined thirty-eight males (mean age, forty-two years) in a residential treatment program. They were evenly split between experimental and placebo groups. The experimental group took vitamin supplements (three capsules per day), each containing vitamins C (333 mg) and E (66 IU), niacin (333 mg), and vitamin B_6 (66 mg) for three weeks. The regimen produced a significant decrease in depression and lowered anxiety as compared to the placebo group. Other studies have shown similar reductions in three to six months of vitamin therapy, but this study demonstrated the effectiveness of megavitamin doses in producing clinical improvement in as little as *three weeks.*[21]

It is something of a chicken-and-the-egg situation when you look at nutrition and alcoholism. Does heavy alcohol use cause malnutrition, or does malnutrition lead to alcoholism? We say that the answer is "yes" to both. We think nutritional deficiency is a major cause of alcoholism, perhaps the chief cause. At the very least, malnutrition makes alcohol abuse much harder to stop or even prevent. In infancy, a vitamin deficiency may predispose toward alcoholism in later life. One very interesting study found that infantile vitamin K treatment was associated with "significantly lower rates of alcohol dependence and fewer symptoms of problem drinking" in adulthood.[22]

Alcoholism almost guarantees nutritional inadequacy, and nutritional inadequacy almost guarantees depression and/or anxiety. Every nutrient is important to a healthy person, and all the more so for an alcohol user. For example, alcoholic depression is associated with inadequate folate intake, and it responds to folic acid and vitamin B_{12} supplementation in much higher than the typically recommended quantities.[23]

Niacin deficiency disease (pellagra) is also much more common in alcoholics.[24] One of the prime symptoms of pellagra is depression. Similarly, classical thiamine (vitamin B_1) deficiency disease (beriberi) can be found in alcohol abusers.[25] Acute scurvy, the most serious and clinically obvious vitamin C deficiency disease, can also be seen in alcoholics.[26] Listlessness and depression are signs of both beriberi and vitamin C deficiency. Minerals as well as vitamins are depleted in alcoholics, especially magnesium[27] and calcium.[28] In fact, there is scarcely a vitamin or mineral that alcoholism does not negatively impact.

If alcohol abuse can lead to multiple nutrient deficiencies, it also creates the symptoms associated with those deficiencies. These may manifest differently from person to person, but psycho-pathological symptoms and neurological damage are the rule, not the exception, with prolonged nutrition deficiency. "The classic signs of vitamin deficiency only occur in states of extreme depletion and are unreliable indicators for early treatment or prophylaxis of alcoholic patients at risk. Postmortem findings demonstrate that thiamine deficiency sufficient to cause irreversible brain damage is not diagnosed antemortem in 80–90 percent of these patients. . . . As the condition of the patient misusing alcohol progresses, damage to brain, liver, gastrointestinal tract, and pancreas continue to further compromise the patient. Decreased intake, malabsorption, reduced storage, and impaired utilization further reduce the chances of unaided recovery."[29]

Malnutrition is the worst side effect of drinking, and the one all too often ignored. All the patience, counseling, and pharmaceuticals in the world will not correct the depression caused by a lack of nutrients. Only a good diet—very rich in nutrients and very low in unhealthy foods like junk food and sugar—can correct the problem. Nutritional supplementation corrects it much faster. One study found that "short-term supplementation with physiological doses of antioxidant vitamins, carotenoids, and trace elements during alcohol rehabilitation clearly improves micronutrient status indicators."[30]

It is interesting how often a healthy diet and a good supplement regimen produces not side effects but rather side benefits. This can be seen in the connection between alcoholism, anxiety, and depression. Alcohol is itself a depressant. Anxious people may drink. Depressed people may drink. So doing, they both get more depressed. Then they drink more, as one alcoholic put it, "not to be drunk, but to avoid being sober." And they get still more depressed. Depression and alcohol can make a deadly combination—either is a major factor in suicide; in concert, they are worse.

When you cure the one, you are a long way to curing the others. Bill W. had formed Alcoholics Anonymous and stopped drinking long before he started taking niacin. He took niacin for his depression, not for his drinking. But high doses of niacin, vitamin C, and other essential micronutrients also help stop the drinking. It is a chicken-or-egg situation, but exactly which is preeminent does not matter. Nutrition stops alcohol abuse, nutrition stops anxiety, and nutrition stops depression. For many people, when you cure one, the others become manageable, or vanish entirely.[31]

ance by taking a lot of just one is like devoting all your baseball practice time to your pitcher. You might get a lot of strikeouts, but if anybody hits one, you are in trouble. No single player has ever won a World Series by himself, and no single B vitamin can do the job that the whole "team" can do.

Vitamin B_6 by itself in doses of 2,000–6,000 mg daily (that's up to 3,000 times the U.S. RDA) can produce side effects and is therefore way too much to take. Very few persons report symptoms on 1,000 mg daily, and only the most rare reports go any lower. When taken with, or as part of, a complete B-complex supplement, B_6 side effects, other than a harmless deeper-colored urine, are virtually unknown.

Zinc

Drinking a lot of alcohol causes zinc (as well as niacin) deficiency.[16] And what's worse, that very zinc deficiency may make it harder to stop drinking the alcohol that caused it.[17] It is a vicious cycle, unless you start taking extra zinc. Supplemental zinc may actually help a person get off alcohol addiction.[18] Zinc also strengthens the alcohol-damaged immune system[19] and increases the ability of the body to properly metabolize alcohol.[20]

A good supplemental dose of zinc is 50–100 mg per day of zinc citrate. Zinc gluconate or zinc monomethionine are also good supplemental forms.

Potential Zinc Side Effects

On an empty stomach, some people will feel a temporary upset with zinc. Therefore, zinc should be taken with a meal. It is very safe even in daily doses of hundreds of milligrams. Very high doses (500 mg or more) over the long term may cause a copper deficiency. Just a milligram or two of copper per day is sufficient to offset this. Multiple vitamins, and copper water pipes in your home, usually provide sufficient copper.

Vitamin B_1 (Thiamine)

In 1897, a prison doctor named Christiaan Eijkman first cured beriberi. Many of his prisoners had the disease. They were fed a diet of primarily polished (milled or white) rice, the stuff so many people eat to this day. Dr. Eijkman fed the prison diet to chickens and observed them to have the same beriberi symptoms. He then fed the sick chickens unmilled, natural (brown) rice, and the birds were cured. He gave whole brown rice to the prisoners, and they were cured as well. All it took was brown rice, and something special in that unprocessed rice.

In 1911, Casmir Funk, a Polish chemist living in London, would discover the first of the special "somethings" in the outer, usually wasted rice hulls. Because it was a nitrogen compound, he labeled it an "amine"; and since it was vital to health, it was a "vital amine"—a vitamine or vitamin. The name stuck and became a generic designation. Between 1909 and 1916, the Philippines-based American R. R. Williams began curing beriberi in young children with outstanding success. The rice polishings he used were thereafter called vitamin B (for beriberi?) and thought to provide a single essential chemical. Today, known to be a team of vitamins, the B-complex vitamins are water-soluble, indispensable, and generally not stored by the body. Thiamine proved to be the cure, and the only cure, for beriberi. It is designated as vitamin B_1 (one of its parts is a *thiazole* ring, and it is a *vitamin*, hence the name).

Thiamine is activated by thiamine pyrophosphate (TPP) to form a coenzyme needed in glucose oxidation to either get energy from glucose or to produce storage fat (lipogenesis). Without thiamine, these do not occur. Hence the fatigue and wasting away typical of beriberi. The mineral magnesium is another essential cofactor in this process.

Thiamine is not stored in tissues. You need it every moment of every day, and it plays a crucial role in carbohydrate metabolism, pregnancy, lactation, and muscular activity. Less well known is that more thiamine is needed in tissues during a fever. A deficiency of thiamine may produce indigestion, severe constipation, insufficient hydrochloric acid secretion, edema, weakened heart muscle and heart failure, reduced alertness, fatigue, and apathy. A long-standing inadequate or marginal thiamine supply may cause severe neurological effects, most significantly nerve irritation, diminished reflex response, prickly or deadening sensations, pain, damage to or degeneration of myelin sheaths (the fatty nerve cell insulation material), and ultimately paralysis.

Beverage alcohol is ethanol (C_2H_5OH), a simple carbohydrate much like sugar, supplying lots of energy and no other nutrients. Thiamine is needed for carbohydrate metabolism. Extra carbohydrates, including alcohol, require extra thiamine. Because alcohol is filling, it displaces more nourishing foods in the diet, causing malnutrition and specifically causing thiamine deficiency. So, the heavy drinker is much less likely to get even the usual dietary amount of thiamine at a time when he or she needs much more. Still worse, alcohol causes poor absorption and poor utilization of what B vitamins there are. A deficiency of thiamine and magnesium in alcoholics may be a factor in the development of delirium tremens (DTs) and alcoholic encephalopathy.[32] Thiamine-deficiency nerve damage can result in the DTs and hallucinations.

The U.S. RDA of thiamine is only a milligram or two, which is not even close to being enough. A very strong case can be made for 25–65 mg per day, even for nonalcoholics. The heavy drinker's poor diet, plus ensuing alcohol damage and increased thiamine need, points to an optimum B_1 intake of several hundred milligrams a day.

Potential Thiamine Side Effects

Oral supplementation with thiamine, even in extremely high does, is exceptionally safe. There are virtually no reported side effects from B_1 except for very rare hypersensitivity reactions to thiamine injections.

Vitamin C (Ascorbic Acid)

Vitamin C improves and accelerates the metabolism of the toxic byproducts of alcohol and has also been shown to be effective against hepatitis.[33] Vitamin C plays a major role in physical medicine, especially in the treatment of cancer. In mental illnesses, it is not as relevant as are the B vitamins, but due to its antistress properties, it is advantageous to use 1–3 grams (1,000–3,000 mg) daily.

Much higher quantities of vitamin C, on the order of 10,000–40,000 mg per day or more, may be needed. The indication of body saturation is bowel tolerance, or the amount of vitamin C that causes loose stools. Why so much? Beverage alcohol (ethanol) is chemically similar to methanol (windshield washer fluid) and propanol (rubbing alcohol), both of which are poisons. In quantity, vitamin C is an antitoxin.[34] High doses of vitamin C chemically neutralizes the toxic breakdown products of alcohol metabolism, and vitamin C increases the liver's ability to reverse the fatty buildup so common in alcoholics. Researchers have shown that vitamin C protects the liver. Even doses as low as 500 mg daily helps prevent fatty buildup and cirrhosis.[35] A total dose of 5,000 mg of vitamin C per day appears to actually flush fats from the liver.

Potential Vitamin C Side Effects

Vitamin C is remarkably safe. The major side effect when large doses are used is loosening of the stools. This is not real diarrhea as there is no pain or cramps. But if it occurs, the dose should be decreased to below this level. The jingle to remember is "Take enough C to be symptom free." That is, enough to feel good, but not enough to produce loose stools. As mentioned above, this is called "bowel tolerance."

Other Important Nutrients

Essential Fatty Acids (EFAs)—It is now corroborated by research that essential fatty acids are therapeutic for a large proportion of psychiatric conditions, including schizophrenia and mood disorders. Researchers such as Dr. David Horrobin have specifically connected alcoholism with a special need for EFAs.[36] Gamma-linolenic acid may help prevent fatty liver, an all-too-common disease of alcoholics.[37] Essential fatty acids are found in abundance in flaxseed oil and in the nonliver fish oils. Fish liver oils also contain some, but they also contain vitamins A and D, which are not always needed as much as EFAs are. Typical dose: 1,000–3,000 mg taken three times daily.

Chromium—The mineral chromium, deficient even in most healthy people, is almost certainly wanting in the alcoholic's diet. Chromium improves your body's sensitivity to insulin, so you can do more with less of it. Remember that alcoholics consume huge amounts of simple carbohydrates. The last thing an alcoholic's body needs would be insulin-resistant cells. We recommend a daily dose of 200–400 mcg chromium nicotinate (also known as chromium polynicotinate). Other forms of chromium will also work, although perhaps not as well.

L-Glutamine—The amino acid L-glutamine has long been considered useful for helping to break an alcohol addiction. Its value was first demonstrated over fifty years ago in animal studies.[38] Studies with humans have shown that L-glutamine improves brain function in alcoholics, resulting in improved sleep, decreased anxiety, and a reduced craving for alcohol.[39] Typical dose: approximately 3,000 mg daily taken in divided doses between meals.

Lecithin—Lecithin makes up about a third of your brain by dry weight. Lecithin also provides choline, which your body can make into the neurotransmitter acetylcholine. Acetylcholine produces a feeling of well-being and self-control, and it is therefore wanting in most alcoholics. Additionally, lecithin is lipotrophic, which means it can help move fats in the body. The fatty liver condition so common in alcoholics is likely to improve with lecithin supplementation. Typical dose: 2–5 tablespoons daily.

COMPATIBILITY WITH MEDICATIONS

This nutrient program is entirely compatible with any medication. Most of the alcoholics we have seen are already heavily medicated and have been on treatment for some time. The medication should be maintained at the same level and the above program is introduced. It may take a month or two before the nutrient program begins to show evidence of its effect. If the medication is reduced too early, the patient may relapse. But after two months, if the patient is better or shows some evidence that the drugs are having a stronger effect, then they are very carefully and slowly decreased, consistent with good psychiatric practice. The aim is to have the dose of medication so low that the patient is well with no side effects; in many cases, if treatment is started early enough, the dose may be decreased to zero.

Orthomolecular therapy does not mean that medication cannot be used. It is aimed at recovery no matter what has to be used, provided that the treatment is nontoxic and allows patients to improve. Modern medication is very powerful, and if the dosages are not decreased, the drugs can cause a drug-induced psychosis and the therapeutic effect of the nutrient program may be missed entirely. Nutritional improvement becomes apparent after the toxic effects of the drugs are minimized by decreasing drug doses.

EXERCISE AND STRESS REDUCTION

Exercise, as you might guess, helps reduce alcohol cravings.[40] Stress reduction through meditation has also been demonstrated to reduce alcohol use.[41] Exercising more, and practicing a stress reduction technique, have zero harmful side effects, and countless side benefits. Try them and see.

THE BOTTOM LINE

Persons truly seeking to kick alcohol need to eat more fiber and more vegetables, and take a lot more vitamins. They also need to avoid sugar and eliminate junk food. People who do not want to change their diet and do not want to change their lifestyle are tempted to ask doctors for a pill instead. There is no such thing as monotherapy for addiction.

This program works. I (A.W.S.) have personally observed how charitably dispensed vitamin supplements help street people and how wheat germ (a natural but modest source of B vitamins, among other good things) helps those in prison. Remember, many people want to stop drinking but can't unless they have the bodily strength to do so. Since alcohol hurts the body, we have to first fight back with vitamins, and then we can reach our goals. Don't tell someone to stop drinking—empower them to stop drinking. Studies confirm it: good eating stops bad drinking.

CHAPTER 5

RESULTS OF VITAMIN TREATMENT

Bill W. (William Griffith Wilson), cofounder of Alcoholics Anonymous (AA), was the first person to test the value of niacin (vitamin B_3) in the treatment of AA members. This treatment had been developed by Dr. Humphry Osmond and I (A.H.) in our work with schizophrenics in Saskatchewan, Canada. During early pilot studies, we observed that patients with the double diagnosis—schizophrenia and alcoholism—responded well to treatment with vitamin B_3, especially niacin. I had already become convinced from my clinical studies that to help the schizophrenic component of the double disease would be very helpful, simply because this removes one of the major stressors from these patients.

One of my patients was both alcoholic and schizophrenic, but whenever she stopped drinking with the help of AA, she began to suffer violent auditory hallucinations. When she began to drink again, the voices disappeared. She was faced with a terrible dilemma: she would either have to remain alcoholic, with all that entailed, but free of voices, or she would have to remain abstinent but suffering from these voices. She tried abstention several times with no luck. I started her on niacin (1,000 mg after each of three meals), and within a few months, when she stopped drinking, the voices did not come back. After that, she became a valued member of the first Schizophrenics Anonymous group I organized in Saskatoon, Canada.

From Bill's informal group of thirty people, ten were improved at the end of one month, another ten at the end of two months, and the rest had not been helped after three months. This was one of the first indications that niacin would be helpful for alcoholics who were not drinking but who still were not well and suffered from a variety of mood disorders, including depression, fatigue, and anxiety. Niacin, in combination with other B vitamins, had proven to be lifesaving for alcoholics suffering from delirium tremens (DTs), so we were not surprised with Bill's confirmation.

Encouraged by the support from doctors in AA, Bill planned on distributing the information as widely as possible. He discussed this with the International Board of AA in New York, which disapproved. Looking on this treatment as part of medicine, they did not think that Bill should become involved in medical matters. They were correct that it was medical, but even now very few doctors consider the use of vitamins as a practical part of medicine. Bill was not deterred and decided to do this on his own, bypassing the board. Some of the letters from the medical members of his board showed that they disapproved vehemently.

BILL W.: A GREAT ADVOCATE OF VITAMIN THERAPY

Bill wrote three communications to AA's physicians called *The Vitamin B₃ Therapy*, the first distributed in 1965, the second in 1968, and the third in 1971.[1] However, he did not think that the words *niacin* or *nicotinic acid* (niacin's original chemical name) would capture enough attention. One evening, he asked me about this, and I told him that niacin had previously been designated as vitamin B_3, because it was the third water-soluble B vitamin to be identified. So Bill began to use the designation vitamin B_3, even though by then the use of letters to identify vitamins was being discontinued in the medical world. But Bill's use brought it back and it is today called B_3, even in the most conservative medical literature.

Bill strongly promoted niacin as a nutritional treatment. He thought that AA should take the following actions:

- Fund and advocate research on niacin.

- Encourage its members to take niacin and improve their nutrition (eat whole foods and reduce intake of excessive sugars, refined carbohydrates, and caffeine).

- Advocate that all AA physicians as well as any physicians treating alcoholism should advise their patients about vitamin therapy.

Unfortunately, AA rejected these recommendations then and evidently continues to reject them. We now know that niacin decreases the mortality from the DTs, and niacin reduces acetaldehyde levels from the metabolism of alcohol, thus reducing oxidative stress.[2] A whole-foods diet, along with a decreased intake of sugar and refined carbohydrates, is necessary to boost long-term recovery rates. Bill's recommendations, if adopted, might have alleviated a great deal of suffering.[3]

By January 1968, in his second communication, Bill was encouraged by an explosion of interest. He recorded that total niacin sales increased from almost none in 1965 to 24,000 orders in 1967. Bill wrote, "This rapidly accelerating interest has been most surprising, considering the institutional apathy and lack of knowledge which has been the rule for many years past." Had Bill lived another ten years, the use of niacin in alcoholics would have been well established. However, his important contribution will not die. Over the years, I have seen a large number of members of AA who chose to use niacin, and it has been extraordinarily successful.

Bill reported on a Texan member of AA who learned about massive niacin or niacinamide therapy from another member and was dramatically and rapidly relieved of a chronic depression. He then prepared a large mailing on the subject to physicians and AA members in his area. A regional vitamin wholesaler soon received large numbers of B$_3$ orders from Texas. These types of stories continued to be repeated. Bill spoke to an old AA friend in the New York area who had endured years of acute depression. Vitamin B$_3$ relieved his condition, and he began to recommend the vitamin to fellow AA sufferers. In consequence, he estimates that some 400 people in his vicinity are now using B$_3$. The same phenomenon repeated itself in Norway, Holland, Finland, Germany, England, Australia, and South America.

FIRST MENTAL HEALTH CENTER USE OF B$_3$

In March 1966, psychiatrist David Hawkins, M.D., founder of the former North Nassau Mental Health Center, in Manhasset, Long Island, and his colleagues adopted the B$_3$ therapy program. Because of the safety of niacin, they felt there was nothing to lose by trying the Hoffer-Osmond treatment on schizophrenics in their care, as well as alcoholics with schizophrenia and numerous nonschizophenic alcoholics suffering depression, insomnia, anxiety, and exhaustion. Many of these alcoholics were sober because of AA, but still felt miserable. Many others were too emotionally or physically ill to achieve sobriety through AA or any other approach. After more than two years of B$_3$ experience, the results were surprisingly good—indeed, amazing.

In the first five years, they treated over 4,000 patients with the megavitamin approach, including approximately 600 alcoholics. The great majority showed marked improvement. "Most of them could be called recovered," noted Dr. Hawkins, "if we define 'recovery' as the ability to function satisfactorily in the community with little or no professional help. The alcoholics, of course, must also be able to maintain their sobriety."

Dr. Hawkins conducted the first major investigation of orthomolecular treatment for alcoholics both with or without schizophrenia. He began using this approach for schizophrenia in 1966 and his open study was intended to derive clinical experience using a biochemical treatment approach for recovering alcoholics.

THE HOD DIAGNOSTIC TEST

The Hoffer-Osmond Diagnostic (HOD) test is a very useful diagnostic tool, developed initially for use with schizophrenics. It is based on an organic hypothesis of schizophrenia: that the intensity of the psychotic or neurotic manifestations would be revealed by the degree that the senses (sight, hearing, taste, smell, etc.) were affected. Using responses from normal individuals as a baseline, a questionnaire (the HOD test) was created to reveal the kind and level of perceptual distortions experienced by patients. It consists of a series of cards with statements relevant to the perceptions, which the patient answers as "true" or "false." Here are a few statements from the HOD test:

- When I look at people they seem strange
- My thinking gets all mixed up when I have to act quickly
- Pictures appear to be alive and to breathe
- I can read other people's minds
- People's faces seem to change in size as I watch them
- I often hear or have heard voices talking about or to me
- People watch me all the time
- I often hear my thoughts inside my head
- I now become easily confused
- People's eyes seem very piercing and frightening
- Sometimes I feel very unreal
- I have to be on my guard with friends
- There is some plot against me
- At times my mind goes blank
- At times some other people can read my mind
- Some foods that never tasted funny before do so now
- I find that past, present, and future seem all muddled up

HOD testing consumes very little time and can be accurately scored by almost anyone. A normal score was calculated to be under 40, but it was found that seriously ill schizophrenics could have scores ranging from 75 to as much as 150! Plus, the severity of the illness in its various mental and emotional manifestations could be readily diagnosed.

Patients are routinely given the HOD test before being placed on the B_3 therapy and other supportive medications. Two to three months later, when the patient again answers the identical questionnaire, his or her score has often made a noticeable drop toward normal. If B_3 is withdrawn at this time, after a similar period it is found that the score often returns to the higher figure, and the patient is as sick as ever.

HOD testing has revealed a large incidence of schizotendencies among people who had not been previously diagnosed using ordinary psychiatric methods. For example, of 200 alcoholic admissions in a hospital in Saskatchewan, Canada, 33 percent were shown to be alcoholics with schizophrenic tendencies. Some other hospitalized alcoholic groups have shown a higher percentage than this, although some have been lower. This suggests that the incidence of undiagnosed schizophrenia or schizotendencies among alcoholics is many times greater than had been previously demonstrated, although many psychiatrists have long suspected the existence of this relationship.[4]

The HOD testing kit, along with full directions, can be obtained from: Behavior Science Press, 3710 Resource Drive, Tuscaloosa, AL 35401. Telephone: 800-826-7223, 205-758-2823, or 205-247-3134.

The study consisted of 315 patients diagnosed with schizophrenia who applied for treatment at an outpatient clinic. The diagnosis was confirmed by the Hoffer-Osmond Diagnostic (HOD) test or diagnostic psychological tests. Seventy of the 315 patients (22 percent) had alcoholism as well as schizophrenia. Most patients were chronic, with either the paranoid or undifferentiated type. Eighty-nine percent of the patients had had previous treatment or hospitalization.

After the diagnosis was confirmed, the patient and/or their family was told that the patient was suffering from schizophrenia. When possible, the patient was also encouraged to attend either Schizophrenics Anonymous (SA) or recovery group meetings. Each patient was then given the following:

- Niacin or niacinamide (minimum daily dose of 3,000 mg and a maximum dose of 12,000 mg)

- Ascorbic acid (4,000 mg per day)

- Pyridoxine or vitamin B_6 (200 mg per day for the first month, then 50 mg daily)

- A phenothiazine drug, given for its antischizophrenic effect and/or tranquilizing properties

In this way, the patient's illness was seen as being primarily a medical problem with psychological and social consequences. The patients were seen about once a month. They were not asked to stop smoking, but they were encouraged to get daily physical exercise. They were also advised to keep caffeine to a minimum and most were put on a hypoglycemic diet.

The improvement rate was surprisingly high, especially considering that many of the patients had already had previous and often extensive treatment elsewhere. Infrequent patient visits, spaced at increasing intervals, were quite sufficient for most patients. The treatment protocol was economical and easily within reach of every family. The use of the HOD test clarified the diagnosis for many patients and the medical staff as well, increasing their understanding of the illness. The presence of the same perceptual distortions in multiple patients worked against a simplistic psychodynamic formulation of the disease.

There were only mild side effects from high-dosage B$_3$ treatment. Niacin and niacinamide were found to be less effective in adult schizophrenics with childhood or adolescent onset. The overall improvement rate was 71 percent, and the best response was obtained in the seventy patients with schizophrenia plus alcoholism. This was attributed to the fact that the majority of these patients also went to both AA and SA. Of the patients who were currently sober, only a few failed to show improvement of the schizophrenia. The clinical manifestations of schizophrenia abated in the patients in response to biochemically oriented treatment.

An Integrated Treatment Program

The program at the North Nassau Mental Health Center evolved into an integrated treatment system that included the following:

- An outpatient treatment center that specializes in treating schizophrenia, alcoholism, and other perceptual illnesses, including megadoses of vitamins, notably B$_3$.

- A hospital facility that accepts referrals with the understanding that vitamin treatment methods will be used.

- A halfway house and day-care activities for those recovering from the illness, focusing on rehabilitation in an orthomolecular patient regimen.

- Alcoholics Anonymous and Schizophrenics Anonymous groups, including continual supervision of medication and diet.

- Working with community doctors who are skilled in megavitamin therapy and the HOD test.

The improved treatment methods have shown some valuable advantages, according to Dr. Hawkins. The need for hospitalization has been reduced 80 percent. Psychiatric treatment time (per patient) has dropped 80 percent. The need for extensive psychotherapy has been greatly reduced, and constructive family involvement has greatly increased. This has drastically lowered both diagnostic time and treatment costs.

Among alcoholic patients, three problems cropped up again and again, which led to "falling off the wagon" or prevented full emotional recovery despite sobriety:

- The use of the hypnotics, barbiturates, or tranquilizers—Taking even small amounts of these substances seriously interferes with the patient's sobriety and brings about subtle alterations in mental and emotional function.

- Functional hypoglycemia (hyper-insulinism) or low blood sugar—This accounted for many failures to recover. Hypoglycemic alcoholics felt better as soon as they were taken off sugars and sweets and started taking B_3. Correction of hypoglycemia eliminated depressions, feelings of tension, anxiety, and recurrent desires to drink in the majority of patients.

- The presence of multiple perceptual distortions (revealed by the HOD test)—These malfunctions have a profound effect on mood, judgment, and the ability to discriminate reality. In some patients, the HOD score was so high as to give the alcoholic symptoms of schizophrenia. Though hallucinations are common during DTs, many such alcoholics continue to have hallucinations long after they have stopped drinking.

The orthomolecular approach concentrates on searching for biochemical abnormalities in patients and correcting these before dealing with any psychological approaches. "We have found that the great majority of our patients have biochemical and metabolic problems, conditions which have been extremely important in preventing any worthwhile recovery," states Dr. Hawkins. "In a very sizeable percentage of patients, once these abnormalities are corrected, rapid progress and recovery is the usual outcome."

FETAL ALCOHOL SYNDROME

If the sins of the parents are often visited upon their children, this applies particularly to fetal alcohol syndrome. The metabolic derangement caused by the mother's use of alcohol during pregnancy surely is also present in the fetus, and they are left with a major problem for which there appears to be no simple and effective treatment. I (A.H.) successfully treated several of these children with a high-dose multivitamin program, emphasizing niacin (vitamin B_3). The results with these patients have shown that this is the right approach and, of course, it will not do any harm.

L.R., born in May 1994 and seen in September 2004, had been diagnosed with fetal alcohol syndrome. Her great aunt took care of her. She had been neglected, and she continued to have major difficulty in focusing. L.R. would have to be asked the same question over and over again, she learned slowly, and she suffered from mood swings. She was hypervigilant and physically aggressive toward her younger sister. Dexedrine made her much worse and caused severe nightmares and visual illusions. Ritalin, which was not as toxic as the Dexedrine, did not have any therapeutic effect.

Her aunt placed her on a dairy-free diet, which was followed by major improvement. I added niacin (100 mg after each meal), ascorbic acid (500 mg after each meal), essential fatty acids, and a multivitamin. L.R. did not like the niacin flush (the harmless side effect that sometimes accompanies taking niacin), so the B_3 was changed to inositol niacinate (a nonflush form), 500 mg three times daily. When seen ten months later, L.R. was almost normal. Because she had lost so much valuable learning experience, her aunt planned to have her go to a special school where she would be able to receive more attention from her teachers. She was cheerful, relaxed, and well on the way to complete recovery.

Her younger sister was born in March 2001. She was examined at the same time as L.R., although she appeared to be normal. It seemed likely that fetal alcohol syndrome might express itself later on. She was started on a similar program and, when she was last seen, she too showed major improvement.

All of Dr. Hawkins's patients responded to a megavitamin regimen, and many patients on the niacin therapy reported a greatly diminished desire to drink, in addition to improvement in their other symptoms.

"The theory behind the megavitamin approach is that the megavitamins correct the abnormal breakdown of adrenaline into toxic byproducts, which are the cause of the perceptual alterations and the elevated HOD score," states Dr. Hawkins. "Practically speaking, when we take patients off harmful drugs, correct their hypoglycemia, and then place them on megavitamins, sometimes with the addition of one of the phenothiazine [antipsychotic] drugs, remarkable recoveries are often the result. It is clinical results rather than theory which concern us."

FIRST ALCOHOLIC TREATMENT FACILITY TO USE B$_3$

In early 1966, after seeing a copy of Bill's first communication, Austin Ripley, director of the Guest House in Lake Orion, Michigan, a center for the rehabilitation of alcoholic priests, began to employ B$_3$. After Mr. Ripley's medical staff consulted with Dr. Osmond and I and saw our positive reports, they recommended that the B$_3$ therapy be added to the Guest House treatment program. All priests were first HOD tested and then placed on 3,000 mg or more of B$_3$ daily. The HOD test had shown that the alcoholic priests were 40 percent perceptually affected.

Mr. Ripley contacted priests who had remained sober by

means of the Guest House program plus membership in AA, but who continued to suffer from emotional instability. One of these was a Jesuit priest who Bill referred to as "Father Joe." He was a professor of philosophy at a major university and had a lifelong history of depression. After two years of sobriety, Father Joe's depressions were actually worse and almost continuous in nature. Unable to teach for long stretches of time, his life work was threatened.

Father Joe's score on the HOD test was highly abnormal. He was prescribed vitamin B_3 (3,000 mg daily); this helped, but he still was not well. The dose was raised to 6,000 mg and eventually to 9,000 mg daily. On the higher dose, he recovered completely. Father Joe went on to start a Schizophrenics Anonymous group in the New York area, including both nonalcoholic schizophrenics and AA members. The original group expanded so rapidly that it split into two groups of over sixty members each.

FATHER JOE'S MODEL OF SCHIZOPHRENICS ANONYMOUS

Of the original group in Father Joe's Schizophrenics Anonymous (SA), which numbered over 100, 30 percent were alcoholic-schizophrenics and AA members, while the rest were nonalcoholic schizophrenics. SA's program was based on the principles of AA, along with any necessary medical treatment and adherence to somes simple health rules.

To begin physical recovery, the SA member was urged to see a doctor who comprehended the vitamin therapy regimen— megadoses of vitamins B_3 and C, plus vitamins B_1 and B_6, and any necessary antipsychotic medications if medically indicated. "From a regular association with his doctor, the patient achieves a solid conviction of the physical nature of his disease," stated Father Joe. "He readily comes to know the various aspects of the disease as they affect him. Through his doctor, he learns the importance of rest, exercise, high-protein diet, avoidance of coffee, Cokes, excessive carbohydrates and sugar, etcetera." The SA therapeutic process cannot be wholly successful without a physician's assistance and encouragement.

Each member learns how to self-administer the HOD test, so he or she can check on progress as well as any relapses. In this way, it is possible to detect early signs of symptoms returning because of stress, anxiety, forgetting to take the vitamins, improper diet, and so on. All of these "slips" show up very quickly on the test.

When the person begins to feel better physically, he or she joins a regular SA group, which emulates the AA "steps" program. This helps the person accept the disease and acknowledge the responsibility for repairing the damage it has brought. "Through sharing his experience with other members, he finds the hope that these corrective principles can and will restore him to health and sanity," states Father Joe. "He is able to communicate, often for the first time, with the other members of his group who have endured his experiences and afflictions." The person learns that by helping others, he is helping not only himself, but also his family and society—a spiritual bonus of inestimable value. The SA member is able to mature emotionally, learning to cope with fears and feelings of hostility and isolation. "Thus, he builds on to his physical and psychological recovery a creative and constructive structure of spiritual values."

Schizophrenics Anonymous Member Stories

John D.

My first experience with drinking came at the age of seventeen, at which time I had my first drink, my first drunk, and my first blackout. When I graduated from high school, I was a weekend drinker and the first serious incident of my drinking occurred. I was in a barroom fight, and because of the damage to my face, I was unable to go to work for a week.

After six months, I volunteered for the draft. The Korean War was going on at the time and the thought of being out on my own appealed to me. By the time we got overseas, I was drinking heavily, frequently skirting serious trouble only by a hair. After twenty months of active duty, I was sent to an army psychiatrist. He said he could help me if I chose to stay in the service, but I was ashamed and accepted a general discharge.

After my return home, I was unable to go back to work right away. Instead, I just idled around the house. I remember one time going downtown in the city during the day and being terrified by the crowds and the traffic. I know now that the schizophrenia was beginning to make itself felt. Finally, I started working and enrolled in college at night. After two years, during which time the weekend pattern of drinking became a way of life, I tired of the routine, felt a desire to get into newspaper work, and quit work and college within two weeks.

I went to Florida for a rest, and I remember trying to stay away from a drink for the first three or four days. This worked for a while, but eventually the loneliness caught up with me and I went into a bar for one drink. The next day, when I came out of the blackout, I found I had only my bus ticket left and seventy-five cents in change. I got back to New York and fortunately in two weeks got a job on a paper. I felt happier then, even though relations at home were strained to the point of long periods of silence becoming commonplace after my drinking bouts.

The changes in my personality were becoming more pronounced. The shyness was taking greater hold of me. I was frightened of the idea of sex and found it painful and embarrassing to be in the company of women when I was sober. However, within a year, I met a girl and found myself engaged. I say "found" because the engagement just seemed to happen. But before too much time went by, I was drinking more and more heavily and frequently in front of the girl. She gave me back the ring, and I left New York to work on New Jersey papers. The jobs got better through the years but the drinking got worse. I was thrown out of one apartment because of my drinking, and a little later I had an automobile accident while drunk on the job.

I was about 28 and the pattern of isolation had become pronounced. I was back living with my family. I worked nights, and consequently the only time I had for recreation was weekends. Invariably, I was drunk on weekends and now found myself getting drunk more frequently during the week. After four years in New Jersey, I decided to try for a job in New York again and I located one. However, prior to my switching jobs, I was hospitalized, this time for a cerebral concussion sustained in a bar fight.

When I started my new job I was terrified. It was a day job and the office was huge. I found the shyness had become such a block that I dreaded going into the office every day. More and more frequently, the drinking was becoming a daily occurrence. After a year-and-a-half of this existence, I got drunk one day at my parents' house, blacked out, and on the way home fell down a flight of subway stairs. Two months after my discharge from the hospital for this episode, I was out on a date and for some reason found myself being repulsed by the drink I held in my hand. I felt as if I were chained to alcohol and no longer had control of it. I decided then to see if I could stay away from a drink for just twenty-four hours.

I did stay away and decided to see if I could do it for two days. Gradually, I built up to a week and then two weeks. But I was becoming more and more frightened. I was afraid to drink now because I thought if I did I would be killed in a blackout. Finally, after almost a month and a half of this, I was having dinner with a friend one night and he broke his anonymity, told me he was in AA, and suggested I give it a try. Within two weeks, I went to my first meeting. Fortunately, I identified from the first night.

I began going to meetings regularly and within three months met the man who was to become my sponsor. I also discovered the Closed Step meetings, and suddenly sobriety began to take on a new meaning for me. The program was making more sense, and I began to experience a great deal of comfort. Very slowly, a new pattern of life began to emerge and even though I was still subject to rapid mood changes, going from deep depression to elation within minutes, and was still subject to violent fits of deep hostility, I was enjoying life more.

However, when I approached my second AA anniversary, I began to notice that the odd feelings of mood changes were becoming more and more pronounced and that I seemed to be very ill at ease at many meetings. I began to think this was to be my lot for the rest of my life, despite the fact that other men who came into the program about the same time I did seemed to be enjoying a happy sobriety.

Finally, my sponsor met Drs. Abram Hoffer and Humphry Osmond and heard their definitions of schizophrenia. He suspected that several of us whom he had been trying to help might also have this illness. I was given the HOD test and was diagnosed schizophrenic. I began taking massive doses of vitamin B_3 and the other vitamins (C, E, B_1, and B_6) and a phenothiazine. Within three months of taking niacin, I suddenly found myself free from the staggering fatigue from which I used to suffer. I felt more alert and more interested in daily life. Within six months, I began to notice a release from the strange thoughts that had been with me all my life. These frequently took the form of bizarre sexual images and gave me a lot of trouble.

I also noticed I enjoyed AA meetings much more than previously. We also formed a group called Schizophrenics Anonymous, and I found a great deal of relief in attending these meetings. I began to pay much more attention to the schizophrenia than to the alcoholism. I soon discovered a train of thought that had me thinking perhaps my real trouble all the time had been schizophrenia and not alcoholism. Fortunately, through the grace of God, I realized the danger in this rationalization and was able to accept that I was *still* an alcoholic as well as a schizophrenic.

Today, I find a great deal of help at both AA and SA. Because of the chemical help I received from niacin, I am able to get much more from AA than I used to. My life is becoming more and more normal and stable and I do not suffer nearly as much from depression, paranoia, or the sudden mood changes.

Vincent C.

Because I am a schizophrenic and recovering, thank God, my experience may be of value to others. As far back as I can remember, it was extremely difficult being around people whom I did not know very well and to whom I could not express my feelings. My self-image was degrading and I was usually a victim of fear. School was a most torturous experience, particularly mathematics. It was laborious to retain knowledge and to continue in the process of learning.

I was reared a baptized Roman Catholic and the training received became a source of pain, stress, and confusion. There is no blame with my religious profession. Most of the time I suffered from introversion, however, at other times I became grandiose. Depression and elation were the mainstays of my life. Rarely was I ever comfortable with myself. An occasional expression of humor helped me to prevent complete insanity.

A significant change came after my introduction to alcohol. The wonderful changes that took place through excessive consumption were a source of definite release. "I am," so I thought, "free again from the prison of myself." Consequently, I resorted to alcohol every opportunity I had. Many times I passed out and suffered blackouts, but this I thought was a small price for the feelings I enjoyed while drinking. Drinking became the hub of my existence. My experiences with alcohol unmistakably pointed to the fact that I am alcoholic.

I am twenty-seven years old and sober three years. I drank excessively for ten years, starting out on this path when I was fourteen. I went through many friends, many jobs. However, I did graduate from high school. At a point of time the alcohol no longer was effective in releasing me from my miserable and distorted existence. I became very frightened. I did not wish to live, and I could no longer consume alcohol safely. I felt completely lost and useless to myself and others.

Through a friend, I became a member of Alcoholics Anonymous. At my second AA meeting, I met my sponsor, who was to show me the way out and how to live. I tried very hard to work the AA program. The longer the distance from the last drink, the worse I seemed to be getting physically and emotionally. The perception distortion of the sense images, the suspicion, the lack of belief, depressions, and paranoia became most severe without alcohol. I remained in my apartment most of the time and very rarely answered the phone or used it. Job situations became increasingly painful and, consequently, I kept losing jobs when I thought there should have been more stability in my life. The "locked-in" feelings deepened and cut off communication. After a year and a half of sobriety, a breakthrough came.

My sponsor became acquainted with Dr. Hoffer, who had been involved in research into the nature and causes and recovery from schizophrenia. I came to know of Dr. Hoffer's therapy for schizophrenics—massive doses of niacin (vitamin B_3) and ascorbic acid (vitamin C). I came to know of the effectiveness of Schizophrenics Anonymous, which follows the model of AA except for the emphasis on the disease of schizophrenia.

I took the HOD test. Now I know I am a schizophrenic, have been, and will continue to be even though recovered. I am also alcoholic, permanently addicted to alcohol, despite a day-to-day recovery. This knowledge brought me great relief and made clear to me many childhood disturbances. There was a great deal of work to do, however.

It was recommended as an essential step that I consult a doctor who prescribed the vitamin therapy for schizophrenia, and Dr. David Hawkins became my medical advisor. Because the HOD test score was 157—very high in perceptual distortion, paranoia, and depression—the doctor prescribed, in addition to B_3 and C, vitamin B_6 (pyridoxine) and a phenothiazine.

The periods of the recovery process were quite varied, and often painful. Regular physical exercise was strongly suggested: I selected to swim four times a week. My diet changed from heavy carbohydrates to high protein and some fat. Rest consisted of eight hours each day and one morning sleep-in until noon.

My artistic ability to paint helped a great deal and, in addition, I am taking lessons on the guitar. Pleasant colors and sounds help enormously to reduce my anxiety.

I am very well now, one year after I began the "chemotherapy." There is continuous serious need for self-imposed discipline. Meals must be on time. The prescribed chemotherapy has to be taken with regularity and at the times indicated. All the areas of this simple but total therapy are interdependent. Physical well-being helps to lead to emotional maturity, and both of these set the stage for spiritual growth.

In closing, I have never in my life felt as well as I do now—a world of reality completely new to me, filled with enthusiasm and challenge. The HOD score is below 30 now.

THE FRUSTRATIONS OF FINDING HELP FOR ALCOHOLISM

(This is a condensed version of the following paper: Lee, Mickey M., Ed.S., and Humphry Osmond, M.R.C.P., F.R.C.Psych. "John's Saga: A Case Study of Alcoholism in the 70s." *J Orthomolecular Med* 5:3 (1976): 222–227. Used with permission.)

John, a 25-year-old psychologist working on his Ph.D., was an alcoholic. He came from a poor family in the coal mining regions of northwestern Pennsylvania. He is the oldest of five children, both parents being alcoholics, and his mother is probably a chronic schizophrenic. There is also a long family history of alcoholism on both sides of the family.

In his particular subculture, it is the custom for younger males to drink heavily as this is held to be a sign of manhood. This environmental pressure, combined with the possibility of being genetically predisposed toward alcohol, John began to drink early and heavily. At sixteen, he started heavy beer drinking, which served as an escape from his home and became a way of gaining prestige among his peers. After entering college, this drinking pattern continued. John received encouragement for drinking in his fraternity where being able to hold your liquor was considered an affirmation of masculinity.

He began to reflect very seriously upon his personal and family history after an uncle died of alcoholism at the age of thirty-five. His temperament led him to seek help from a psychologist/friend and teacher, who had an extensive background in psychoanalysis. Although the professor was highly competent, his cultural and personal inclinations led him toward a bibulous form of psychoanalysis. Consequently, when John left undergraduate school, he was still drinking beer almost as heavily as ever, but had in addition acquired a taste for wine. While this improved his social repertoire, it did not allay his growing worries about developing alcoholism.

Once away from his psychotherapist, John began a series of increasingly desperate attempts to get help for his drinking problem. His first step was to seek more orthodox assistance. He turned to Alcoholics Anonymous. However, knowing little about the many different kinds of AA groups, he stumbled upon a very traditional, pious, and older AA group, mostly in their forties and fifties. He found the rituals and customs of this particular group tedious and soon left discouraged.

He continued to look for help and moved in the direction of medicine. He had heard that Antabuse (disulfiram) helped many alcoholics and proceeded to research it in a systematic way. It seemed to him that since he had a strong and growing desire to stop drinking, but was under a variety of external pressures to continue, Antabuse might be the extra incentive needed to stop. He therefore approached several doctors and received some totally unexpected and discouraging responses. Several of the doctors, confusing models, applied the moral instead of the medical model.

John entered an Ed.S. program in school psychology. At this time, he received extensive training in behavior modification techniques, which were espoused as a panacea for a great variety of problems. Since one of John's professors was an authority in this field, John approached him concerning the possibility of doing some type of behavioral therapy with him. The answer he received was curt and direct. "Because prognosis for alcoholism is so poor, I avoid it." John was confused and distressed, for being aware that he had a potentially fatal illness, he had done everything that an intelligent person could do.

By May 1975, John was still drinking and beginning to study for his Ph.D. at a southern university. He realized by now that his drinking was beginning to interfere with his academic/social functioning and this made him increasingly anxious and depressed. John was becoming very frustrated. He had tried for four to five years to obtain help, and for the previous two years had intensified his efforts, but had failed to discover even the vestige of an answer to his grave problem. Becoming seriously depressed and seeing no hope, he began to consider suicide.

Because of John's training, temperament, and personal involvement, we hoped that we would give him immediate reinforcement in the form of hope, further alternatives, and a greater understanding of his condition. The following ideas were suggested:

- Minor tranquilizers to reduce his withdrawal symptoms.

- Changing his diet (reduction of carbohydrates and increased protein consumption), increasing his exercise, and possibly using megavitamins.

- Once his withdrawal symptoms had been alleviated, the use of Antabuse as a means of establishing and maintaining a new pattern of behavior.

- The possible use of psychotherapy because it deals especially with enlarging one's knowledge of one's own temperament.

John's approach to his illness was sensible and systematic. Indeed, it is quite unusual to find a young man who is so interested in and aware of the implications of his condition. However, as this story shows, for the best part of five years John was not in the least benefited by what one might have thought would have been a notable asset, that is, his training as a psychologist. He discovered that many professionals appear to be intimidated or annoyed when a patient deviates from what they believe to be the traditional patient role. John received no encouragement and a good deal of bad advice.

John is currently in excellent health. The changes in diet combined with megavitamin therapy have increased his feelings of optimism and self-esteem. Although he occasionally has the desire to drink, he feels that the use of Antabuse provides him with an external incentive needed to establish himself as a nondrinker with accompanying behavioral patterns.

CONCLUSION

Since the time of these early reports, every physician who has used orthomolecular treatment for alcoholism obtained the same results. Unfortunately, the few clinical trials that have been conducted, with one exception, made no attempt to repeat this earlier work. The exception is the study Bill W. encouraged by Dr. J.R. Wittenborn and financed by the National Institutes of Mental Health (NIMH).[5] Dr. Wittenborn released two reports. In the first, he used a combination of early and chronic patients and he could then find no difference. But when this was pointed out to him, he reviewed his data and separated the two groups. He then found that with his twenty-four subjects who were early, the vitamin group showed a 70 percent response rate compared to a 35 percent response rate in the placebo groups. This is exactly what the earlier report showed. He published the revised findings in his second report. The American Psychiatric Association seized on his first paper with great enthusiasm and totally ignored his second report, even though both were published in the same journal. The psychiatric establishment did not want any treatment to be positive unless it involved drugs only. This, to a large degree, is still their attitude to this day.

CHAPTER 6

THE CONTROVERSY OVER PSYCHEDELIC THERAPY

Psychedelic drug treatment for alcoholism was first investigated in the 1950s, showing some positive results for a select group of alcoholics. Nevertheless, it remains a controversial therapy to this day. In the interest of comprehensiveness, we present information here on the therapeutic uses of psychedelics for alcoholics.

"MIND MANIFESTING"

The term *psychedelic* was created by Dr. Humphry Osmond in Saskatchewan, Canada, and first announced at a meeting of the New York Academy of Sciences in 1957. He described the use of hallucinogens like LSD (lysergic acid diethylamide) to induce an experience that could be enormously helpful in changing that individual thereafter. It is important to know that it was the experience that changed the person and that the particular drug used to induce it did not matter much.

This is how the concept was discovered. Dr. Osmond and I (A.H.) had treated a few alcoholics in the hospital, admitted with delirium tremens (DTs). About 20 percent of these patients died from this condition. We had been exploring LSD and mescaline, and later adrenochrome and adrenolutin, as a way of getting to understand better what it was like to be schizophrenic. The experiences were not identical with schizophrenia for many reasons, but they were as close as one could get without actually becoming schizophrenic. The DTs is not a pleasant experience, but sometimes alcoholics who recovered from them did not drink any more. It was described as "hitting bottom." But hitting bottom naturally was very dangerous.

It occurred to me in 1952 that we might use the LSD experience as a safe way of inducing a delirium-like experience to show patients what might happen to them if they kept on drinking. Dr. Osmond thought this was a good idea. Several alcoholics who had been committed for treatment under Dr. Osmond's supervision agreed to take the LSD. After five or six patients had been treated, Dr. Osmond and his research psychologist concluded that these experiences did not resemble DTs and that the patients, rather than being terrified, enjoyed the reaction. This happened so frequently that Dr. Osmond was convinced this was a new phenomenon—he coined the word *psychedelic,* which means "mind manifesting."

We then changed our orientation: instead of using the experience to frighten patients that they might get DTs, we hoped to use the psychedelic experience to encourage them not to drink. Instead of giving them a psychotomimetic experience, we wanted to give them the psychedelic experience.

We began to treat more and more alcoholics in three psychiatric wards of a general hospital and in two mental hospitals. Approximately 2,000 alcoholics were treated over a five-year period, and about 40 percent were helped by psychedelic therapy and did not drink any more. They had all been admitted, which meant they had failed every known treatment. The results were published in a number of publications. We no longer considered it research.

Not every alcoholic was treated this way and we had firm criteria:

- Every treatment was voluntary with informed consent.

- Schizophrenia was not treated.

- They were treated in a hospital and only by doctors and nurses who had been educated in the proper use of these drugs.

As a result, we had no prolonged reactions. If they were not out of the reaction after a few hours, they were given niacin, either intravenously or by mouth, which would terminate the reaction in about ten minutes.

The psychedelic treatment went into hibernation. The psychedelic explosion that followed soon made it impossible to continue, and by 1960 we were no longer treating anyone. This was a pity as so many had been helped. Many years later, I encountered some of these patients and they were still abstinent.

A FACILITATOR

I do not by any means recommend that every alcoholic should be treated using psychedelics. The majority of alcoholics do not need it and will respond to orthomolecular treatment. But some who cannot find the incentive to change their behavior may benefit.

For example, Carl was a very severe alcoholic admitted to a hospital in Saskatoon. He was a likable psychopath and was always very pleasant and agreeable to every treatment suggestion, except that he did not stop drinking. He was so skillful in getting his favorite drink that he would get drunk while a patient in the hospital. I thought he would be ideal for psychedelic treatment, as his prognosis was so poor and this would be an ideal test of the treatment. Carl agreed and was given the usual small dose of LSD. Nothing happened, and I later learned that he was certain it would not have any effect on him "because of his superior brain." I asked him if he would try it again, and the second time I gave him a larger dose. Again, nothing seemed to happen, except that he was uncomfortable and tense. However, when I debriefed him the next morning, he told me that around 11 A.M., which was usually when they started to have the most intense experience, he suddenly had a vision of God, who wiggled his finger at him and said, "Carl, no more." He never drank again.

The treatment should be reserved for alcoholics who have not responded to any other treatment, and it should always be voluntary. It does not have to be LSD; mescaline, dimethyltryptamine (DMT), ibogaine, and other substances can create the same kind of experience. The drug is not the treatment—it is a facilitator.

Recently, there has been new attention to this unusual approach to alcoholism. Says one author: "Today, after a thirty-year hiatus, this research is gradually being resumed, and there is renewed interest in . . . psychedelic research, the therapeutic use of LSD in the treatment of alcoholism."[1] Psychedelic therapy was used with some success for autism in the 1950s and 1960s.[2] Hallucinogens have also been found to be effective to help treat obsessive-compulsive disorder[3] and depression.[4] Psychedelic treatment was controversial at the time, and remains so today.

CHAPTER 7

STOPPING TOBACCO SMOKING AND CAFFEINE USE

TOBACCO ADDICTION

When actor and heavy smoker Yul Brynner (1920–1985) was dying of lung cancer, he was asked on television if he had any words to offer about smoking. He looked straight into the camera and said, "Just don't do it." Advice that can save 450,000 lives a year is good advice indeed. In the United States alone, tobacco kills fifty-one people *each hour.* Of course, the tobacco industry spends over $11 million every single day on advertising to encourage this. Those who have tried know that stopping smoking is easier said than done. Nine out of ten smokers say they'd like to quit, and nine out of ten who do quit used no special technique at all—they take Yul Brynner's advice and just stop doing it.

It works even better with a special technique: spray vitamin C into the back of the mouth and throat each time you want a cigarette. Yes, vitamin C sprayed into the mouth during cigarette smoking gradually reduces the craving to smoke. By the end of one study, smoking behavior was either reduced or stopped completely.[1] Isn't it a wonder that we have never been told about this amazingly important research?

So, where can you buy vitamin C spray to help stop smoking? We have no idea, but we think you are better off making your own, fresh, every day. Vitamin C (ascorbic acid) powder is cheap, and you can probably find a sprayer at the dollar store. Mix as much of the crystalline vitamin C as will dissolve in an ounce of water and spray the back of your throat every time you want a cigarette. The vitamin C technique not only helps you stop smoking, it also helps control hunger cravings and reduce that old nicotine withdrawal weight-gain syndrome.[2]

If you do not have an extra spray bottle lying around, you can just gargle with it. Or use chewable vitamin C tablets, or drink the vitamin C solution, or just take a lot of vitamin C tablets orally. Because vitamin C is a weak acid (like carbonated soft drinks), rinse your mouth with water afterward. You can also buy buffered vitamin C powder or use nonacidic chewable tablets. All these will help you stop smoking and reduce food cravings at the same time.

Many people are familiar with the serenity prayer: "Give me strength to change the things I can, serenity to accept the things I cannot, and wisdom to know the difference." Well, smoking is something we *can* take personal control over.

Vitamin Therapy for Nicotine Addiction

An alternative approach to standard methods of nicotine replacement therapy (NRT)—gum, inhalation, nasal spray, transdermal patch—may be the oral administration of vitamin B_3 (niacin or niacinamide). That's because niacin is chemically similar to nicotine, and nicotine might occupy niacin receptor sites in the central nervous system (CNS), creating a niacin deficiency. Thus, the calming effects of cigarette smoking may actually be the result of nicotine occupying these niacin receptor sites, making it possible to wean smokers off nicotine by administering niacin.[3]

Jonathan E. Prousky, N.D., professor of clinical nutrition at the Canadian College of Naturopathic Medicine, in Toronto, reported using niacin or niacinamide in seven patients with a nicotine addiction (1,500–3,000 mg per day). He found that vitamin B_3 significantly reduced the cravings for nicotine by approximately

50 percent. In two cases, just using B_3 enabled the patients to wean off cigarettes comfortably within 2–3 weeks. The other patients continued to smoke, but their cravings for cigarettes were considerably reduced and their intakes of cigarettes were halved as a result of the vitamin B_3 treatment.[4]

Thus, the addiction to and cravings for nicotine might exacerbate a vitamin B_3 deficiency and stimulate a biological need to have niacin receptor sites occupied. Nicotine addiction and other conditions such as alcoholism may belong to a category of diseases known as NAD deficiency diseases.[5] The deficiency of NAD results in unwanted behaviors and addictions geared toward filling NAD receptor sites. We think alcoholism is a good example of an NAD deficiency disease.

NAD stands for nicotinamide adenine dinucleotide, which is made directly from vitamin B_3. It is the active form of the antipellagra vitamin niacin. NAD is one of the most important coenzymes in your body, involved in many oxidation-reduction reactions. Electron-rich, it is called NADH; electron-poor it is called NAD. Both activate a number of enzymes. NADH is essential for energy production; without it, we would not get energy from the food we eat. NAD activates alcohol dehydrogenase and acetaldehyde dehydrogenase, two enzymes that detoxify alcohol, breaking it down into carbon dioxide and water.

"The principle treatment," states Dr. Prousky, "is the administration of optimal amounts of vitamin B_3 in order to cover the NAD receptor sites and shut off the vicious addiction-withdrawal cycle." Alcohol consumption increases the formation of acetaldehyde, which forms morphine-like compounds that fill NAD receptor sites in the brain and temporarily shut off withdrawal symptoms. When these receptor sites become unoccupied or unbound, withdrawal symptoms occur and the craving for alcohol begins once again. Researchers have found that it is possible to stop the addiction-withdrawal cycle by substituting optimal amounts of niacin for alcohol.[6] This leads to a reduction of drinking behaviors, cravings, and withdrawal symptoms.

Nicotine addiction, like alcoholism, is a disease where NAD deficiency is central to the addiction-withdrawal cycle. It should also be noted that acetaldehyde is found in tobacco smoke as well; it has very addictive opiate effects within the central nervous system.[7] In the same way that niacin reduces acetaldehyde concentrations from alcohol, vitamin B_3 might reduce acetaldehyde produced from tobacco smoke and diminish nicotine cravings. "Vitamin B_3 might, in fact, be the best alternative method of treatment for nicotine addiction," concludes Dr. Prousky.

CAFFEINE ADDICTION

A popular series of 1950s magazine advertisements for decaffeinated coffee depicted husbands so afflicted with "coffee nerves" that they were more like beasts than men. One such cartoon illustration actually showed the husband in a cage, raging and railing against his terrified family from behind bars. But it's not funny. Caffeine, the most common and most unrestricted of stimulant drugs, has diverse and adverse effects on the human body.

I (A.W.S.) recall my first pharmacologically memorable encounter with caffeine. I was in my teens, in London, and spotted an elderly lady going down a long flight of steps with a cane in each hand. It was the classic Boy Scout opportunity, for it truly looked as if she was going to topple over any second. I caught up with her and helped her across the street. Across the street turned out to be the location of her hotel, and she graciously invited me, the touring Yankee, to have coffee with her in the hotel's elegant sitting room. She turned out to be a brilliant conversationalist. Hours went by, and in that time I downed eight cups of coffee. I felt just great.

Back at my hotel that night, I went to sleep, sort of. It was not long before I awoke, my eyes wide open. I tried to close them, and they instantly leapt open again. It was as if my eyelids were on springs. This went on for some time, as I lay there and figured out, eventually, what transpired—I'd had about 1,000 milligrams of caffeine, and it was working.

The Familiar Stimulant

Caffeine, an alkaloid methylxanthine, is incredibly well absorbed when taken orally: 99 percent of it goes straight into your body. It passes easily through the blood-brain barrier. It is a central nervous system stimulant, a skeletal muscle stimulant, and a cardiac stimulant that induces hypoglycemia,[8] agitation, insomnia, altered mental states, rigidity, tremors, and seizures. The familiar is often the last thing to be suspected, and nothing is more familiar than caffeine. It is consumed worldwide at an estimated 120,000 tons per year.

Caffeine is said to have a half-life in your body of three to seven hours. Not only does that vary among people, it also needs a comment. Using five hours as the average, this means that ten hours after consumption, 25 percent of the drug (at least) is still in you. Women on the birth control pill take twice as long to metabolize caffeine as women who are not. And some persons are vastly more sensitive to caffeine than others. It's not just coffee that's the caffeine culprit: tea, chocolate, many pain relievers, and soft drinks contain caffeine.

Children and Caffeine

An increasingly large number of children—nearly three-quarters of all children over the age of six months—are having that same xanthine blast as mom and dad.[9] The Center for Science in the Public Interest has reported that about half of all children drink soda pop, and those between ages six and eleven drink nearly a pint a day. Of the seven best-selling soft drinks, six have caffeine in them.[10]

A concerned parent wrote: "Our 11-year-old son became extremely strange and looked almost insane, pulled pranks, and barely remembered what he had done. We were worried, as he had always been happy and a model student, devoted to music and hard work. It all disappeared. At first, we did not know what was causing the sudden deterioration in his personality. We thought about teenage hormones. We then discovered that he consumed a bottle of soda pop or a can of energy drink on the way home from school every day. I searched the Internet and discovered the large amounts of caffeine in the soft drinks he consumed, and I read about caffeine's effect on the brain. We eliminated all the caffeine-containing foods and drinks (as far as I know) from his diet and now he seems almost back to normal."

Lendon H. Smith, M.D., frequently said that if your child craves something, it's probably not good for him or her. Caffeine is a stimulant, not as powerful as Ritalin or amphetamines, but a stimulant nonetheless. When, exactly, does "just say no" to drugs begin? By law, nicotine use is prohibited until age eighteen; alcohol use is prohibited until age twenty-one. And yet we know of no age restrictions on caffeine.

If there were an age restriction on caffeine, it would have to start even before birth. Caffeine crosses the placenta, causing an overactive fetus. The developing baby gets as much as the mother. Babies so affected cry more and sleep less. Women who drink more than a cup of coffee every day are only half as likely to conceive as those who drink less than a cup a day.[11] Furthermore, if a pregnant woman drinks 2–3 cups of coffee each day, she is more likely to have a premature baby or a full-term infant with low birth weight.

Strategies for Eliminating Caffeine

Some people should not consume any caffeine. Sensitive persons may experience a profound cerebral allergy, manifesting as an actual caffeine psychosis.[12] Ruth Whalen learned this the hard way. She suffered for over twenty years from various psychoses that, she discovered, were cured when she eliminated caffeine.

She wrote *Welcome to the Dance* (Victoria, BC, Canada: Trafford Publishing, 2005) to tell her intensely personal story and to take a medically comprehensive look at just how severe caffeine's negative effects can be. She narrates how she lost twenty-seven years of her life to unrecognized caffeine-induced psychosis. And then she cured it, not by taking a pharmaceutical drug but by refusing to take a common dietary drug. If you (or someone you care about) is a caffeine user and life is a mess, we encourage you to read her book before things get any worse. If a person is psychotic, bipolar, or suffers from obsessive-compulsive disorder, perhaps the answer is not to take more drugs, but to take fewer. Start by stopping caffeine.

In fairness, it needs to be said that for a stimulant drug, caffeine has relatively few other negative long-term effects. Miscarriage or low birth-weight babies, heart attack, elevated blood pressure, benign breast lumps, panic attacks, and lower academic performance may result from habitual, maintained caffeine use. With caffeine consumption equivalent to 7–10 cups of coffee a day for an extended period of time, there could be observable and perhaps permanent damage to the rhythm of the heartbeat.

If you "need" your morning cup of coffee, you are, if ever so civilized, addicted to caffeine. The proof is in the stopping: physical withdrawal symptoms confirm a physical dependence. How do you stop caffeine intake without the withdrawal headaches? Here are some helpful suggestions:

- Vitamin C reduces caffeine withdrawal symptoms, especially the headache. It also reduces cravings for drugs, including nicotine and even narcotics. As Ewan Cameron, M.D., and Linus Pauling reported in their book *Cancer and Vitamin C,* "Five ascorbate-treated patients who had been receiving large doses of morphine or heroin to control pain were taken off these drugs a few days after treatment with vitamin C was begun, because the vitamin C seemed to diminish the pain to such an extent that the drug was not needed. Moreover, none of these patients asked that the morphine or heroin be given to them—they seemed not to experience any serious withdrawal signs or symptoms."[13] Regarding proper dosage, take enough C to be symptom free, whatever the amount may be. Although it normally can take a couple of months to get over a caffeine habit, high antitoxic doses of vitamin C can greatly speed the process.

- To alleviate the psychological need or dependence, substitute a cup of something else for your morning coffee. "Postum," herbal tea blends, hot water and lemon, or hot cider are all good choices. Enjoy the ritual and comfort of preparing and drinking a steaming mug of caffeine-free "something else." Even decaffeinated coffee is a good start.

- What about regular (nonherbal) tea? While there is caffeine in regular tea, it is only roughly half that of coffee. Tea also contains some antioxidants, which are good for you. Both green tea and black tea leaves are picked off the same plant, *Camellia sinensis*. The difference is that green tea is not aged (fermented), whereas black tea is. Uncrushed, unoxidized green tea leaves are healthier for you, but both types naturally contain caffeine. A 5-ounce cup of average-brewed tea has roughly the same amount as a 12-ounce caffeine-containing soft drink.

- Homeopathy may be of help.[14] Years ago, a national advice columnist published a reader's letter claiming that eating a pinch of tobacco before smoking a cigarette reduced the amount of smoking a person did. Maybe it was due to the bad taste or a fear of mouth cancer. Or maybe it was the principle of homeopathy, which may be colloquially explained as "the hair of the dog that bit you." Homeopathic *Tobaccum* 6X (a harmless microdilution of tobacco) might be a more gum-friendly way to try this idea. Perhaps homeopathic unroasted coffee, *Coffea Cruda* 6X, might be worth trying for caffeine addiction.

CHAPTER 8

ORTHOMOLECULAR SUPPORT DURING WITHDRAWAL AND DRUG OVERDOSE

Addicts have to be withdrawn very carefully, with skill and tolerance for the discomfort they go through during the withdrawal process. The difficulty and time required depends not only on the drug to which they have become addicted but also on their nutritional state. With all addictions, attention should be given to the physical health of the patient. Specifically, this means that nutrition must be ensured and the correct vitamins should be given in optimal doses (not the usual low vitamin doses). The nutritional regimen needed to get through the withdrawal will vary considerably.

Alcoholics and sugar addicts need similar programs. I (A.H.) have found that sudden withdrawal, "cold turkey," works best for these addicts. I have seldom seen an alcoholic who can gradually discontinue alcohol. Researchers have found a few alcoholics who, treated with niacin along with alcohol, could gradually stop drinking. For the treatment of delirium tremens (DTs), it is best not to use drugs if they can be avoided.

Addiction to heroin, morphine, and other narcotic drugs can be treated with very large doses of niacin, very large doses of vitamin C, and amino acid drinks. They can be withdrawn in a few days or weeks. Antidepressant drugs should be withdrawn very slowly and carefully. The withdrawal symptoms are not as dramatic as with alcohol and street drugs, but they may last much longer. Few doctors are fully aware of how addictive anti-depressants are. Since they are seldom any better than placebo, according to recent well-publicized studies, it is a shame they are given to patients at all. It may take weeks or months of slowly decreasing doses, and these patients have to be given a lot of support as they are going through withdrawal. The causes of their depression must be determined and treated—these are usually food allergies and the need for nutrients. The worst withdrawal problems are with atypical antipsychotic drugs.

The basics of safe withdrawal are attention to food and the use of nutrients in optimum amounts, lots of support and time, and treatment of the underlying disease that caused the addiction in the first place. Not everyone who is sick becomes addicted, but it is very rare for anyone who is healthy to do so. The ideal treatment is the same for all addictions: the patients must be treated so they become free of all drugs, including prescribed ones.

AN INTENSIVE HOLISTIC APPROACH

Researchers Alfred F. Libby and Irwin Stone found that by using very high doses of niacin and vitamin C, addicts were able to get off heroin in seven days without the usual withdrawal symptoms.[1] Addicts suffer from severe metabolic dysfunctions and are, in fact, very sick, so we again emphasize that any solution to addiction must focus on first restoring total health.

Humans in general, and drug addicts in particular, are affected by humankind's genetic inability to manufacture the enzyme L-gulonolactone oxidase (GLO), which is needed to synthesize vitamin C from blood glucose. This causes hypoascorbemia (chronically low blood vitamin C levels). It is basically an error of carbohydrate metabolism, which means that almost all humans are suffering from subclinical scurvy. Most people manage to survive this handicap, staying alive on very low dietary quantities of the vitamin. It is a house of cards at best, easily shaken and knocked down by any severe stress to the body. Under stress, humans require an astounding 30,000 to 100,000 milligrams or more of vitamin C per day to regain health.[2]

Addicts generally begin their introduction to the drug culture at an early age, often beginning with tobacco, marijuana, alcohol, and barbiturates and then moving on to harder drugs such as cocaine and narcotics. The weekend "high" escalates into a daily habit from which they can't escape. Each of these stresses further depletes the already very low body stores of vitamin C.

On drugs, the addicts lose their appetite for food, which leads to severe protein and vitamin malnutrition. All the chronic addicts in the Libby and Stone study suffered from low levels of amino acids, the building blocks of proteins. Thus, an addict is suffering from hypoascorbemia-Kwashiorkor syndrome, a type of malnutrition. The treatment proposed by Drs. Libby and Stone is an intensive holistic approach to correct the genetic and nutritional dysfunctions. By fully correcting the nutritional problems, addicts can come off heroin or other drugs without withdrawal symptoms. After a few days on the regimen, appetite returns and they start eating voraciously, and they also have restful sleep.

For the therapy, the narcotic intake is stopped, and the addict is given the first large dose of vitamin C, high levels of multivitamins and minerals, and a predigested protein preparation (9 tablespoons). This means consuming 25,000–85,000 mg of vitamin C a day in frequently divided oral doses. The program is continued for 4–6 days, and then the dosages are gradually reduced; the maintenance dose is about 10,000–30,000 mg of vitamin C per day. Selection of proper dosage is based on clinical experience and responses of the patient. General improvement in the well-being of the addict is usually rapid, within 12–24 hours after beginning detoxification. One will see improved mental alertness, better appetite, and often surprise from the addict that the treatment is working without the use of drugs. In the pilot study of Drs. Libby and Stone, thirty out of thirty patients were successfully treated using this protocol.

For example, T.G., a 23-year-old male, had been using drugs for ten years. At the time that treatment started, he was supporting a $100-a-day (1970s monetary values) heroin habit. On several occasions, he had tried hospital detoxification programs with methadone and liquid Darvon, but substituting another narcotic for heroin failed to provide relief. His urine was tested for urinary spillover of ascorbate and amino acids and there was none, confirming hypoascorbemia and low levels of amino acids. He was started on sodium ascorbate (25 grams daily in divided 4-gram doses) along with the vitamins, minerals, and protein supplements. After three days, T.G. began eating regular meals. He felt better and began thinking more clearly and having more restful sleep. The vitamin C was reduced to 10 grams daily after six days. When last contacted, he had been completely drug-free for three months and had lost his desire for the drug. He was now gainfully employed for the first time in his adult life.

More recently, researchers in Greece reported that with vitamin C in very large doses (300 mg/kg body weight per day), plus very large doses of vitamin E (5 mg/kg body weight per day), half of heroin addicts tested experienced only mild withdrawal symptoms. In the control group, only 7 percent of the cases had mild symptoms. Plus, the vitamin C–treated subjects expressed major withdrawal symptoms in only 10–17 percent of cases, in contrast to the untreated subjects who expressed a major withdrawal symptom in 57 percent of the cases. The results indicate that high doses of vitamin C may ameliorate the withdrawal syndrome of heroin addicts.[3]

Treating Drug Overdose

Drug overdose is a common occurrence because of the variable potency of illicit drugs. Orthomolecular treatment of an overdose acts as an antidote and rapidly relieves the stricken addict. Vitamin C is a very powerful antitoxin.[4] The physician protocol is as follows: if the victim is unconscious, immediately but slowly inject 30 grams (30,000 mg) or more of sodium ascorbate intra-venously; if he or she is conscious and can swallow and retain liquids, give about 50 grams (50,000 mg) of sodium ascorbate, dissolved in a glass of milk.

In one case, a mother brought in her 16-year-old son, who was high on "Angel Dust" (PCP). He was incoherent and totally out of touch with reality. He was given 30,000 mg of sodium ascor-bate mixed in a glass of milk, and within forty-five minutes he could hold a normal conversation. With intravenous vitamin C, recovery time could be reduced to a few minutes.

Why It Works

This reliable, nontoxic therapy has many advantages over the standard way of handling drug addicts. The main antinarcotic effect is due to vitamin C. High levels of ascorbate mimic mor-phine and probably fit into opiate receptor sites in the brain—high levels of sodium ascorbate displace narcotic molecules already attached to these sites. Also, ascorbate is a general detoxicant for many different poisons.

At high intake levels, vitamin C is known to reduce inflamma-tion and act to as a natural antibiotic, antihistamine, and anti-toxin. Surprisingly, it also acts as a powerful pain reliever, a property discovered in the 1970s in Scotland with research on cancer patients. In Great Britain at the time, it was policy to pro-vide terminal patients with any pain relief available, including addictive narcotics such as heroin. The argument was simply that if one were dying anyway, a drug's analgesic value outweighs any drawbacks such as dependency. Five patients treated with vita-min C, who had been receiving large doses of morphine or hero-in to control pain, were taken off the drugs after a few days of ascorbate treatment. The vitamin C seemed to diminish the pain to such an extent that the drug was no longer needed. None of these patients experienced any serious withdrawal symptoms from the morphine or heroin.[5]

The drive for all addicts is the attempt to be relieved of pain and discomfort. Vitamin C takes care of that. Many readers will be puzzled at our assertions. We invite them, and their physicians, to directly consult the references we provide and see for themselves.

CONCLUSION

THE WAY OUT

(A.W.S.) used to teach college courses in jail (no, not as an inmate) as an adjunct professor, part of a certified alcohol counselor (CAC) training program. One course was called "Drug and Alcohol Use and Abuse." As a joke, I've always enjoyed telling people that I taught prisoners how to use and abuse drugs and alcohol. The inmates needed no such instruction: in the two medium-security facilities that I worked at, drug and alcohol use and abuse were, by far, the most common reasons they were in the slammer. There are currently over 2.3 million Americans behind bars, and even with more prisons being built every day, serious overcrowding continues. Most of them are there because of the illegal consequences of abusing drugs and alcohol.

The solution we propose may surprise you—to give nutritional therapeutics a chance. Orthomolecular megavitamin therapy is cheaper, safer, and, in my experience, more effective than drugs or counseling. It is vastly more humane and is immeasurably cheaper for the taxpayer than incarceration, which costs over $55 billion per year.

Incredibly, this knowledge has been available for over fifty years, but it has been overlooked. Bill W., the cofounder of Alcoholics Anonymous, strongly advocated megavitamin therapy for alcoholism back in the 1950s and 1960s, after Dr. Hoffer treated him for depression using niacin. Bill's interest in nutritional therapy has been marginalized and his vitamin recommendations ignored. Half a century later, substance abuse remains an unsolved problem, enormously costly and painful, whether behind bars or in your own neighborhood. Alcoholism and drug addiction, so often portrayed as without cure, can indeed be ended with high-dose nutrient therapy.

THE CHANCE TO BECOME PEOPLE, NOT PATIENTS

In this book, we have shown that alcoholics suffer from a deficiency of several nutrients, and especially from a deficiency of one of the most important B vitamins, niacin (vitamin B3). We think that niacin deficiency in alcoholics is so serious, and the need so pronounced, that it is better termed a *nutritional dependency*. This is probably also true of many of the other addictions.

Some of the evidence was obtained from the early studies by Dr. Hoffer and Dr. Humphry Osmond. A major, and almost universally overlooked, contribution was made by Bill W. after his own research on a small number of alcoholics showed that they also responded to niacin. The subsequent clinical studies, detailed in this book, cemented his view, and the modern evidence adds to this large body of clinical evidence. Every therapist who has used this approach sees the same recovery rates.

It follows that if addicts are sick to begin with, the best treatment is to discover what that sickness is and deal with that first. It is typically a state of clinical *dis*-ease, including discomfort, tension, anxiety, depression, and fatigue, especially in social setting. Symptoms may be ameliorated by pharmaceuticals, which provide some relief but at an enormous cost. Every addict is a diseased person who discovered that street drugs (provided legally and illegally) served them better than prescription drugs, which are used so widely today with so little beneficial effect. Some of these people will find alcohol works best for them.

You have to be sick first before you can become addicted to heroin or cocaine, or addicted to excessive consumption of the sugars. *The underlying problem is poor nutrition.* In every case, the diet is so deficient in the B vitamins that eventually they develop chronic states of pan-nutrient deficiency and nutrient *dependency* that only large doses of the correct nutrients can help. This is why orthomolecular treatment works.

The evidence is in. Even so, today medical evidence is considered adequate only if it is double-blind tested, if it comes out of orthodox medical centers, and if the person making the claim is well known. It does not mean that this standard is better—physician reports provide excellent evidence. In fact, half of the evidence published in medical journals is wrong, and doctors do not know which half that is.

We hope that this book will help educate our society that there are ways of dealing with alcoholism and other addictions that really work and that we do not depend only on what has been tried before, without much success. Legendary comedian W. C. Fields famously remarked that it is easy to stop drinking—he'd done it a thousand times. With orthomolecular nutrition, alcoholics have the chance to become people, not patients. We think that is what Bill W. had in mind all along.

APPENDIX

FINDING RELIABLE INFORMATION ON ORTHOMOLECULAR MEDICINE

NEGATIVE BIAS ON THE INTERNET

Hundreds of millions of people search the Internet daily for health information, but what exactly are they getting? A Google search with the keyword "health" gets you over 900 million results. The United States government holds several prominent spots, such as www.health.gov, www.healthfinder.gov, and www.nih.gov, all U.S. Department of Health and Human Services (HHS) websites. At the U.S. government's Healthfinder website (accessed June 2008), self-described as "your source for reliable health information," it states: "Our website is built on a selection process that begins by evaluating the reliability of organizations as providers of health information. Only after we carefully review an organization do we choose information from its website for our health library." But try a search for "orthomolecular" and you will find *nothing at all.* Your tax dollars pay for such exclusion.

Taxpayers also fund the U.S. Food and Drug Administration (FDA) Dietary Supplements Adverse Event Reporting webpage (www.cfsan. fda.gov/~dms/ds-rept.html), where you can report an illness or injury associated with a dietary supplement. The site actually states that the "FDA would like to know when a product causes a problem even if you are unsure the product caused the problem or even if you do not visit a doctor or clinic."[1] With supplements, perhaps anecdotal evidence is of value after all, provided the anecdotal reports are negative.

One major referral site that has discontinued operations as of October 2007 was HealthWeb (www.healthweb.org), a more or less nongovernmental resource ("a collaborative project of the health sciences libraries of . . . over twenty actively participating member libraries"). HealthWeb, started in 1994, was supported by the U.S. National Library of Medicine (NLM), meaning taxpayer money sponsored it. The project was conceived "to develop an interface which will provide organized access to evaluated noncommercial, health-related, Internet-accessible resources . . . [and] integrate educational information so the user has a one-stop entry point to learn skills and use material relevant to their discipline."[2] We call your attention to the words *noncommercial* and *one-stop* because, at this site, a search for "orthomolecular" also brought up nothing at all.

One of HealthWeb's displayed "nutrition" links led to the "non-commercial" website http:www.ific.org, belonging to the International Food Information Council (IFIC) Foundation. The IFIC's stated mission is to communicate "science-based information on food safety and nutrition" to health professionals, educators, journalists, and others providing information to consumers. But the IFIC is not an impartial purveyor of information—it is supported mainly by the food industry and agricultural interests.[3] This makes the IFIC essentially a lobbyist organization. It claims "partnerships" with such groups as the Food Marketing Institute and the Institute of Food Technologists.[4]

Now, at Google, where there is no evidence of editorial restriction, a search for "orthomolecular" will bring up 390,000 results. While one needs to bear in mind that many of the sites found are anti-orthomolecular, the good news is that more and more are positive.

Still, at many of the largest and most frequented "health" websites, information about orthomolecular medicine is entirely absent. Therefore, when the layman searches for nutritional therapy, they often get false or misleading information from a pharmaphilic (drug-loving) viewpoint. Pharmaceutical medicine's influence on the Internet is very strong, although less dominant than its enormous presence on television and in print media.

On the medical Internet, "reliable" or "carefully selected" seem to mean selection that purposefully excludes orthomolecular medicine. Is there a medical blacklist, and if so, is orthomolecular medicine on it? Terms such as "reliable" and "carefully selected" are meant to imply some kind of objective editing, but when the entire discipline of orthomolecular medicine is excluded, it is in fact censorship by selection.

NEGATIVE BIAS IN GOVERNMENT

The world's largest medical library is biased. The National Library of Medicine indexes most medical journals and makes them instantly accessible through its electronic Medline database. However, the peer-reviewed *Journal of Orthomolecular Medicine* (*JOM*), continually published for over forty years, remains conspicuous by its absence from the library's listings. It publishes high-dose vitamin therapy studies and is read by physicians and scientists in over thirty-five countries. There were 754 million Medline searches in the year 2005, and not one of those searches found a single article from JOM. Some critics accuse NLM of information censorship, which, they maintain, is grossly inappropriate for a taxpayer-funded public library.

Since 1989, JOM has been rejected for Medline indexing five times. This is the decision of a journal review committee selected by NLM. When JOM's editors have tried to clarify just what it is that Medline feels is lacking, they have not received a specific answer. The review committee's score sheet is vague—apparently the JOM's score is not high enough for indexing, but the NLM says it can resubmit and be scored again. Although this has the appearance of open-mindedness, it is a convenient cover for institutional bias.

Of the eight published "critical elements" for Medline journal selection, the tip-off may be this: Medline states that it indexes journals having "articles predominantly on core biomedical subjects," that "scientific merit of a journal's content is the primary consideration," and that they are looking for external peer review. JOM uses external reviewers. Therefore, the real dealbreakers are that JOM is a journal that discusses orthomolecular medicine, a field that the NLM probably considers to be far removed from "core biomedical subjects." And as to "scientific merit," clearly in the eyes of the NLM, JOM lacks scientific merit.

The *Journal of Orthomolecular Medicine* has been published for four decades. It has an editorial review board of physicians and university researchers. And JOM has published papers by prominent scientists, including twice Nobel Prize–winner Linus Pauling, Ph.D.

Medline, to this day (2009), still steadfastly refuses to index the *Journal of Orthomolecular Medicine*. It is reminiscent of a small-town beauty contest: if the contest judges don't like the mayor, his daughter is not going to get a very high score no matter what outfit she wears or what song she sings. If the prosecution picks the jury, the verdict is a foregone conclusion.

To Index or Not to Index

The following papers by twice Nobel Prize–winner Linus Pauling, Ph.D., are not on Medline simply because they happened to be published in the *Journal of Orthomolecular Medicine:*

Rath, M., and L. Pauling. "Solution to the Puzzle of Human Cardiovascular Disease: Its Primary Cause is Ascorbate Deficiency Leading to the Deposition of Lipoprotein(a) and Fibrinogen/Fibrin in the Vascular Wall." *J Orthomolecular Med* 6 (3rd and 4th Quarters 1991): 125.

Pauling, L., and M. Rath. "An Orthomolecular Theory of Human Health and Disease." *J Orthomolecular Med* 6 (3rd and 4th Quarters 1991): 135.

Rath, M., and L. Pauling. "Apoprotein(a) is an Adhesive Protein." *J Orthomolecular Med* 6 (3rd and 4th Quarters 1991): 139.

Rath, M., and L. Pauling. "Case Report: Lysine/Ascorbate Related Amelioration of Angina Pectoris." *J Orthomolecular Med* 6 (3rd and 4th Quarters 1991): 144.

Rath, M., and L. Pauling. "A Unified Theory of Human Cardiovascular Disease Leading the Way to the Abolition of this Disease as a Cause for Human Mortality." *J Orthomolecular Med* 7 (1st Quarter 1992): 5.

Rath, M., and L. Pauling. "Plasmin-induced Proteolysis and the Role of Apoprotein(a), Lysine and Synthetic Lysine Analogs." *J Orthomolecular Med* 7 (1st Quarter 1992): 17.

Pauling L. "Third Case Report on Lysine-Ascorbate Amelioration of Angina Pectoris." *J Orthomolecular Med* 8 (3rd Quarter 1993): 137.

Hoffer, A., and L. Pauling. "Hardin Jones Biostatistical Analysis of Mortality Data for a Second Set of Cohorts of Cancer Patients with a Large Fraction Surviving at the Termination of the Study and a Comparison of Survival Times of Cancer Patients Receiving Large Regular Oral Doses of Vitamin C and Other Nutrients with Similar Patients Not Receiving These Doses." *J Orthomolecular Med* 8 (3rd Quarter 1993): 157.

However, the following papers *are* indexed on Medline; same authors and same topics:

Rath, M., and L. Pauling. "Immunological Evidence for the Accumulation of Lipoprotein(a) in the Atherosclerotic Lesion of the Hypoascorbemic Guinea Pig." *Proc Natl Acad Sci USA* 87:23 (December 1990): 9388–9390. PMID: 2147514 (indexed by PubMed for Medline).

Rath, M., and L. Pauling. "Hypothesis: Lipoprotein(a) is a Surrogate for Ascorbate." *Proc Natl Acad Sci USA* 87:16 (August 1990): 6204–6207. Erratum in: *Proc Natl Acad Sci USA* 88:24 (December 1991): 11588. PMID: 2143582.

Pauling, L., and Z.S. Herman. "Criteria for the Validity of Clinical Trials of Treatments of Cohorts of Cancer Patients Based on the Hardin Jones Principle." *Proc Natl Acad Sci USA* 86:18 (September 1989): 6835–6837. PMID: 2780542.

Pauling, L. "Biostatistical Analysis of Mortality Data for Cohorts of Cancer Patients." *Proc Natl Acad Sci USA* 86:10 (May 1989): 3466–3468. PMID: 2726729.

It is absurd that Medline, which has indexed 116 papers by Dr. Pauling, excludes equally valuable work of his due to where it first appeared. Medline, a service of the U.S. National Library of Medicine, is operated at taxpayer expense. Censorship is unscientific, immoral, and unjust.

HOW TO DESTROY CONFIDENCE IN VITAMINS WHEN YOU DON'T HAVE THE FACTS

"Ladies and gentlemen, welcome to this year's annual meeting of the World Headquarters of Pharmaceutical Politicians, Educators, and Reporters (WHOPPER). Let us get right to the point: many of our members and affiliates have complained about what is, for us, an alarming and dangerous segment of health care—so-called orthomolecular medicine. We wish to assure you, although this therapeutic approach is, unfortunately, very effective in preventing and treating disease, that we will make sure the public will never learn of it. We can say this with considerable confidence, since for over fifty years we have managed to keep virtually all psychiatrists from using niacin to treat schizophrenia; we have kept cardiologists from prescribing vitamin E for heart disease; and we have kept general practitioners from prescribing vitamin C for viral illnesses.

"Yes, it has really been a triumphant half-century. How did we do it? It is really quite easy. Our guiding principle is to keep the public afraid. Any fear will do, but we have been especially pleased with, and therefore recommend instilling, the fear of new strains of flu viruses, fear of vaccine shortages, and, most especially, the fear of vitamin toxicity. Our success with this last one has been nothing short of spectacular. Of course, decades of poison control center statistics show that there have been virtually no deaths from vitamins. You may also know that properly prescribed drugs, taken as directed, kill at least 100,000 Americans annually. Clearly, the last thing we want is for the public to actually figure out that vitamin therapy is tens of thousands of times safer than drug therapy. Therefore, we endorse the following tactics:

"Always demand 100 percent safety and 100 percent efficacy from nutritional therapy. This is particularly effective when, at the same time, you continually remind the public that they have to expect and accept a reasonable amount of dangerous, even fatal, side effects with drug therapy. And if one drug does not work, there is always another, still more expensive drug that might.

"Always give priority to publishing research that portrays vitamins as ineffective or outright harmful. Select the low-dose vitamin study and ignore the high-dose study. Our master stroke is when we criticize low-dose nutrient studies for ineffectiveness, while discrediting effective high-dose studies because they might be dangerous. Remember, pick the one negative vitamin study and ignore the hundreds of positive vitamin studies.

"If a positive megavitamin study is actually submitted to your department, medical society, or journal, reject it on a technicality, and take a year or two to do so. Better still, encourage the authors to publish in the *Journal of Orthomolecular Medicine*. After all, whatever is published there will not be indexed by the National Library of Medicine. Therefore, the public's annual 700 million Medline searches will utterly fail to find it. People cannot read what cannot be located.

"Obfuscation works. Cloud and confuse the issue. Never let the truth stand in the way of a good press release. This we learned from the tobacco industry: if you cannot wow them with wisdom, baffle them with baloney. Remember, with vitamins, always highlight the negative and ignore the positive. Never let the facts get in the way of a good argument (a good argument is one that you win). It's about politics, not health.

"While half the population takes vitamins, fewer than 1 percent of physicians practice orthomolecular medicine. That is a very small minority, so how hard can it be to shut them up? After all, look what we did to Linus Pauling: when he spoke out for vitamin C, we got the entire medical world to openly snicker at the only person in history to win two unshared Nobel prizes.

"Education is a very large number of very small steps. The secret is to keep plugging away, every chance we get. Every time we obscure the facts in the news media or the medical press, it is one additional step toward washing the public's mind clean as a whistle and stamping out nutritional medicine for good. Now, go back to your word processors and get to work. The news media are waiting to hear from you."

Perhaps the World Headquarters of Pharmaceutical Politicians, Educators, and Reporters might be (slightly) fictitious, but the problem is real enough. Negative stories about vitamins indeed have been front-page leads, yet vitamin cures rarely make the evening news. People have heard many a meganutrient factoid, myth, or outright falsehood from their friends, their doctors, or the media. It is truly odd that the public has been warned off the very thing that can help the most—nutritional supplementation. As Ward Cleaver once said to his son, Beaver, on the classic television show *Leave It To Beaver:* "A lot of people go through life trying to prove that the things that are good for them are wrong." Negative reporting sells newspapers and pulls in Internet traffic (the old editors' adage is "If it bleeds, it leads"). Pharmaceutical companies lobby government and feed the media to get the "wonder drug" positive spin, and they have been remarkably successful in so doing, in spite of the 106,000 patients killed annually by their products, even when properly prescribed and taken as directed.[5]

ORTHOMOLECULAR FACTS, NOT FICTION: LOOK AND SEE FOR YOURSELF

Here's one way for anyone to quickly see how safe vitamin therapy is: do an Internet or Medline search for "vitamin death." What will be found is information on how vitamins prevent death. *The Merck Manual* states that there have been two fatalities from vitamin A overdose, spanning many decades of use.[6] There has been a total of one alleged death from vitamin D overdose, due in fact to side effects of medication.[7] We could find no evidence of deaths from any other vitamin. Nonfatal "vitamin danger" allegations are almost entirely without scientific foundation. For example, harmful effects have been mistakenly attributed to vitamin C, including hypoglycemia, infertility, and even the claim that it causes cancer. Vitamin C produces none of these effects.[8]

Since vitamin myths persist, the media are now regularly hearing from orthomolecular medicine. One way is through the Orthomolecular Medicine News Service (OMNS), a project of particular interest to the late Dr. Hugh Riordan, who wanted to promote "an awareness of orthomolecular." Dr. Riordan often said that he wanted "orthomolecular medicine" to be a household word. OMNS seeks to accomplish precisely that. OMNS began full operation in March 2005, and today OMNS press releases are distributed to over 3,000 media outlets worldwide. OMNS asserts and reasserts these positive messages:

- Orthomolecular medicine saves lives.

- The number one side effect of vitamins is failure to take enough of them.

- Vitamins are not the problem—they are the solution.

To receive this wire-service style e-mail without charge, go to www.orthomolecular.org/subscribe.html. All previous OMNS releases are archived at http://orthomolecular.org/resources/omns/index.shtml.

Journal of Orthomolecular Medicine Papers Online

Hundreds of papers from JOM are available for free access on the Internet. Read and decide for yourself if they are worth indexing by Medline.

Linus Pauling on Mental Illness
www.orthomed.org/pauling2.htm
www.orthomolecularpsychiatry.com/library/articles/
   orthotheory.shtml

Linus Pauling Defines Orthomolecular Medicine
www.orthomed.org/pauling.htm

Principles of Orthomolecular Medicine
www.orthomed.org/kunin.htm

Orthomolecular Case Histories
www.orthomed.org/wund.htm

Nutritional Influences on Aggressive Behavior
www.orthomolecularpsychiatry.com/library/articles/webach.shtml

Abram Hoffer on the Megavitamin Revolution
www.orthomolecularpsychiatry.com/library/articles/hoffer.shtml
www.healthy.net/library/journals/ortho/issue7.1/Jom-ed2.htm

Orthomolecular Medicine and Schizophrenia
www.healthy.net/library/journals/ortho/issue7.1/Jom-hk1.htm

Lowering Health Costs with Nutrition
www.healthy.net/library/journals/ortho/issue7.2/Jom-dh1.htm

Abram Hoffer on Vitamin C Deficiency
www.healthy.net/library/journals/ortho/issue7.3/Jom-ed2.htm

Why Vitamin C Megadoses?
www.doctoryourself.com/cathcart_thirdface.html

Vitamin C Therapy
www.doctoryourself.com/mccormick.html
www.doctoryourself.com/levy.html

Vitamin E Therapy
www.doctoryourself.com/evitamin.htm
www.doctoryourself.com/estory.htm

Vitamin D Therapy
www.doctoryourself.com/dvitamin.htm

Gerson Therapy
www.doctoryourself.com/gersonbio.htm

Why Vitamin Supplements
www.doctoryourself.com/replace.htm

Problems with Caffeine Consumption
www.doctoryourself.com/caffeine_allergy.html
www.doctoryourself.com/caffeine2.html

Internet Resources

The complete, free archive of full-text papers from the
Journal of Orthomolecular Medicine
http://orthomolecular.org/library/jom/

Oregon State University's Linus Pauling Institute
http://lpi.oregonstate.edu/

Linus Pauling's 1968 paper on megavitamin therapy,
"Orthomolecular Psychiatry: Varying the Concentrations
of Substances Normally Present in the Human Body May
Control Mental Disease"
www.orthomed.org/pauling2.html

Linus Pauling's 1974 paper on the same subject, "On the
Orthomolecular Environment of the Mind: Orthomolecular
Theory"
www.orthomed.org/pauling.html

Frederick R. Klenner's *Clinical Guide to the Use of Vitamin C*
www.seanet.com/~alexs/ascorbate/198x/smith-lh-clinical_guide_
  1988.htm

C For Yourself
(Information on vitamin C)
www.cforyourself.com

Vitamin C Foundation
www.vitamincfoundation.org/

Ascorbate Web
(A very large number of full-text papers on curing illness with
vitamin C)
www.seanet.com/~alexs/ascorbate

The Vitamin D Council
www.vitamindcouncil.com

Irwin Stone's book *The Healing Factor: Vitamin C Against
Disease*
http://vitamincfoundation.org/stone/

The Biochemical Institute at the University of Texas at Austin
(Contains many of the nutrition papers of vitamin pioneer
Roger J. Williams, Ph.D.)
www.cm.utexas.edu/williams

Townsend Letter for Doctors and Patients
www.tldp.com

Jack Challem's *Nutrition Reporter*
www.thenutritionreporter.com/

Other Works by the Authors

Abram Hoffer—Select Bibliography

Books

Hoffer, A., and H. Osmond. *Chemical Basis of Clinical Psychiatry.* Springfield, IL: Charles C. Thomas, 1960.

Hoffer, A. *Niacin Therapy in Psychiatry.* Springfield, IL: Charles C. Thomas, 1962.

Hoffer, A., and H. Osmond. *How to Live with Schizophrenia.* New York: University Books, 1966. (Revised edition, Kingston, ON, Canada: Quarry Press, 1999.)

————. *New Hope for Alcoholics.* New York: University Books, 1966.

Hoffer, A. *The Hallucinogens.* New York: Academic Press, 1967.

Hoffer, A., H. Kelm, and H. Osmond. *Hoffer-Osmond Diagnostic Test.* Huntington, NY: R.E. Krieger, 1975.

Hoffer, A., and M. Walker. *Orthomolecular Nutrition.* New Canaan, CT: Keats, 1978.

Hoffer, A. *Dr. Abram Hoffer's Guide to the Identification and Treatment of Schizophrenia.* New Canaan, CT: Keats, 1980.

Hoffer, A., and M. Walker. *Nutrients to Age Without Senility.* New Canaan, CT: Keats, 1980.

Hoffer, A. *Nutrition for the General Practitioner.* New Canaan, CT: Keats, 1988.

————. *Orthomolecular Medicine for Physicians.* New Canaan, CT: Keats, 1989.

————. *Vitamin B₃ (Niacin) Update.* New Canaan, CT: Keats, 1990.

————. *Hoffer's Laws of Natural Nutrition: A Guide to Eating Well for Pure Health.* Kingston, ON, Canada: Quarry Press, 1996.

————. *Vitamin B₃ and Schizophrenia: Discovery, Recovery, Controversy.* Kingston, ON, Canada: Quarry Press, 1999.

————. *Common Questions on Schizophrenia and Their Answers.* New Canaan, CT: Keats, 1988. (Reprint, Kingston, ON, Canada: Quarry Press, 1999.)

Hoffer, A., and M. Walker. *Putting It All Together: The New Ortho-molecular Nutrition.* New York: McGraw-Hill, 1998.

Hoffer, A. *Hoffer's A.B.C. of Natural Nutrition for Children.* Kingston, ON, Canada: Quarry Press, 1999.

————. *Orthomolecular Treatment for Schizophrenia.* New Canaan, CT: Keats, 1999.

————. *Vitamin C and Cancer: Discovery, Recovery, Controversy.* Kingston, ON, Canada: Quarry Press, 2000.

Hoffer, A., and M. Walker. *Smart Nutrients: Prevent and Treat Alzheimer's, Enhance Brain Function,* 2nd rev. ed. Ridgefield, CT: Vital Health, 2002.

————. *Healing Schizophrenia: Complementary Vitamin and Drug Treatments.* Toronto, ON, Canada: CCNM Press, 2004.

————. *Healing Children's Attention and Behavior Disorders: Complementary Nutritional and Psychological Treatments.* Toronto, ON, Canada: CCNM Press, 2004.

Hoffer, A., and L. Pauling. *Healing Cancer: Complementary Vitamin and Drug Treatments.* Toronto, ON, Canada: CCNM Press, 2004.

Hoffer, A., and J. Challem. *User's Guide to Natural Therapies for Cancer Prevention and Control.* North Bergen, NJ: Basic Health, 2004.

Hoffer, A., *Adventures in Psychiatry: The Scientific Memoirs of Dr. Abram Hoffer.* Caledon, Ontario: KOS Publishing, 2005.

Hoffer, A., and Andrew W. Saul. *Orthomolecular Medicine for Everyone.* Laguna Beach, CA: Basic Health, 2008.

Papers and Articles

Hoffer, A., H. Osmond, and J. Smythies. "Schizophrenia: A New Approach. II. Results of a Year's Research." *J Mental Sci* 100 (1954): 29–45.

Altschul, R., A. Hoffer, and J.D. Stephen. "Influence of Nicotinic Acid on Serum Cholesterol in Man." *Arch Biochem Biophys* 54 (1955): 558–559.

Hoffer, A., H. Osmond, M.J. Callbeck, et al. "Treatment of Schizophrenia with Nicotinic Acid and Nicotinamide." *J Clin Exper Psychopathol* 18 (1957): 131–158.

Hoffer, A., and H. Osmond. "The Adrenochrome Model and Schizophrenia." *J Nerv Mental Dis* 128 (1959): 18–35.

Osmond, H., and A. Hoffer. "Schizophrenia: A New Approach. III." *J Mental Sci* 105 (1959): 653–673.

———. "Massive Niacin Treatment in Schizophrenia. Review of a Nine-year Study." *Lancet* 1 (1963): 316–320.

Hoffer, A., and H. Osmond. "Treatment of Schizophrenia with Nicotinic Acid—A Ten-year Follow-up." *Acta Psych Scand* 40 (1964): 171–189.

Hoffer, A. "A Theoretical Examination of Double-blind Design." *Can Med Assoc J* 97 (1967): 123–127.

———. "Treatment of Schizophrenia with a Therapeutic Program Based upon Nicotinic Acid as the Main Variable." In Walaas, O. (ed.). *Molecular Basis of Some Aspects of Mental Activity, Vol. II.* New York: Academic Press, 1967.

———. "Safety, Side Effects and Relative Lack of Toxicity of Nicotinic Acid and Nicotinamide." *Schizophrenia* 1 (1969): 78–87.

———. "Pellagra and Schizophrenia." Academy of Psychosomatic Medicine, Buenos Aires, January 12–18, 1970; *Psychosomatic II*, pp. 522–525.

———. "Mechanism of Action of Nicotinic Acid and Nicotinamide in the Treatment of Schizophrenia." In Hawkins, D., and L. Pauling (eds.). *Orthomolecular Psychiatry.* San Francisco: W.H. Freeman, 1973.

———. "Natural History and Treatment of Thirteen Pairs of Identical Twins, Schizophrenic and Schizophrenic-spectrum Conditions." *J Orthomolecular Psych* 5 (1976): 101–122.

———. "Latent Huntington's Disease—Response to Orthomolecular Treatment." *J Orthomolecular Psych* 12 (1983): 44–47.

———. "Orthomolecular Nutrition at the Zoo." *J Orthomolecular Psych* 12 (1983): 116–128.

Hoffer, A., and L. Pauling. "Hardin Jones Biostatistical Analysis of Mortality Data for Cohorts of Cancer Patients with a Large Fraction

Surviving at the Termination of the Study and a Comparison of Survival Times of Cancer Patients Receiving Large Regular Oral Doses of Vitamin C and Other Nutrients with Similar Patients Not Receiving Those Doses." *J Orthomolecular Med* 5 (1990): 143–154. Reprinted in Cameron, E., and L. Pauling. *Cancer and Vitamin C.* Philadelphia: Camino Books, 1993.

Hoffer, A. "Orthomolecular Medicine." In Maksic, Z.B., and M. Eckert-Maksic (eds.). *Molecules in Natural Science and Medicine: An Encomium for Linus Pauling.* Chichester, West Sussex, England: Ellis Horwood, 1991.

———. "How to Live Longer—Even with Cancer." *J Orthomolecular Med* 11 (1996): 147–167.

———. "Orthomolecular Treatment of Schizophrenia." *Complement Med Official J S Afr Complement Med Assoc* 4 (1998): 9–14.

———. "Schizophrenia and Cancer: The Adrenochrome Balanced Morphism." *Med Hypotheses* 62:3 (March 2004): 415–419.

Andrew W. Saul—Select Bibliography
Books

Saul, A.W. *Doctor Yourself.* North Bergen, NJ: Basic Health, 2003.

———. *Fire Your Doctor!* Laguna Beach, CA: Basic Health, 2005.

Saul, A.W., with A. Hoffer. *Orthomolecular Medicine for Everyone.* Laguna Beach, CA: Basic Health, 2008.

Saul, A.W., with S. Hickey. *Vitamin C: The Real Story.* Laguna Beach, CA: Basic Health, 2008.

Papers and Articles

Saul, A.W. "William Kaufman, B_3, and Arthritis." *J Orthomolecular Med* 16:3 (3rd Quarter 2001): 189. Available online at: www.doctor yourself.com/JOM1.html.

———. "In Memoriam: Lendon H. Smith, M.D." *J Orthomolecular Med* 16:4 (4th Quarter 2001): 248–250. Available online at: http://orthomolecular.org/library/jom/2001/pdf/2001-v16n04-p248.pdf and www.doctoryourself.com/smith1.

————. "Taking the Cure: The Pioneering Work of William Kaufman: Arthritis and ADHD." *J Orthomolecular Med* 18:1 (2003): 29–32. Available online at: www.doctoryourself.com/news/v3n16.txt.

————. "Taking the Cure: The Pioneering Work of William J. McCormick, M.D." *J Orthomolecular Med* 18:2 (2003): 93-96. Available online at: www.doctoryourself.com/mccormick.html.

————. "Vitamin D: Deficiency, Diversity and Dosage." *J Orthomolecular Med* 18:3–4 (2003): 194–204. Available online at: www.doctoryourself.com/dvitamin.htm.

————. "Vitamin E: A Cure in Search of Recognition." *J Orthomolecular Med* 18:3–4 (2003): 205–212. Available online at: www.doctoryourself.com/evitamin.htm.

————. "Can Vitamin Supplements Take the Place of a Bad Diet?" *J Orthomolecular Med* 18:3–4 (2003): 213–216. Available online at: www.doctoryourself.com/replace.htm.

————. "Taking the Cure: The Pioneering Work of Ruth Flinn Harrell, Champion of Children." *J Orthomolecular Med* 19:1 (2004): 21–26. Available online at: www.doctoryourself.com/downs.html.

————. "Vitamin Dependency." [Editorial] *J Orthomolecular Med* 19:2 (2004): 67–70. Available online at: www.doctoryourself.com/dependency. html.

————. "Taking the Cure: Natural Health Principles and Principals: Jackson and Macfadden in Dansville." *J Orthomolecular Med* 19:3 (2004): 167–172. Excerpt available online at: www.doctoryourself. com/news/v2 n23.txt.

————. "Medline Bias." [Editorial] *J Orthomolecular Med* 20:1 (2005): 10–16. Excerpt available online at: www.doctoryourself.com/news/v5n10. txt.

————. "Orthomolecular Medicine on the Internet." *J Orthomolecular Med* 20:2 (2005): 70–74. Available online at: www.doctoryourself. com/internet.html.

————. "Vitamins and Food Supplements: Safe and Effective." Testimony before the Government of Canada, 38th Parliament, 1st Session, Standing Committee on Health, Ottawa, Canada, May 12, 2005. Available online at: www.doctoryourself.com/testimony.htm.

————. "Taking the Cure: Irwin Stone: Orthomolecular Educator and Innovator." *J Orthomolecular Med* 20:4 (2005): 230–236. Available online at: www.doctoryourself.com/stone.html.

————, (editor). "Intravenous Vitamin C is Selectively Toxic to Cancer Cells." *Townsend Letter for Doctors and Patients* (December 2005). Available online at: www.townsendletter.com/Dec2005/iv_c1205.htm.

————. "Medline Bias: Update." [Editorial.] *J Orthomolecular Med* 21:2 (2006): 67. Available online at: www.doctoryourself.com/medlineup. html.

————. "Taking the Cure: Claus Washington Jungeblut, M.D.: Polio Pioneer; Ascorbate Advocate." *J Orthomolecular Med* 21:2 (2006): 102–106. Available online at: www.doctoryourself.com/jungeblut. html.

————, (editor). "Vitamin C Prevents and Treats the Common Cold." *Townsend Letter for Doctors and Patients* (June 2006). Available online at: www.townsendletter.com/June2006/vitaminc0606.htm.

Foster, H.D., and A.W. Saul. "AIDS May Be a Combination of Nutritional Deficiencies: HIV Depletes Selenium and Three Amino Acids." *Townsend Letter for Doctors and Patients* (July 2006). Available online at: www.orthomolecular.org/resources/omns/v02n03.shtml and www.alliance-natural-health.org/index.cfm?action=news&ID=236.

Saul, A.W. "Medline Bias." [Editorial.] *Townsend Letter for Doctors and Patients* 277/278 (August-September 2006): 122–123. Available online at: www.townsendletter.com/AugSept2006/medline0806.htm.

————. "Hidden in Plain Sight: The Pioneering Work of Frederick Robert Klenner, M.D." *J Orthomolecular Med* 22:1 (2007): 31–38. Available online at: www.doctoryourself.com/klennerbio.html.

RECOMMENDED READING AND BIBLIOGRAPHY

Recommended Reading

Beasley, J.D. *Wrong Diagnosis, Wrong Treatment: The Plight of the Alcoholic in America.* Dallas: Creative Informatics, 1987.

Dufty, W. *Sugar Blues.* New York: Warner, 1975.

Jacobsen, M. *Liquid Candy: How Soft Drinks are Harming American's Health,* 2nd edition. Washington, DC: Center for Science in the Public Interest, 2005. Free download available at: www.cspinet.org/ new/ pdf/liquid_candy_final_w_new_supplement.pdf.

Ketcham, K., and L. Ann Mueller. *Eating Right to Live Sober.* Seattle, WA: Madrona, 1983.

Larson, J.M. *Alcoholism: The Biochemical Connection.* New York: Villard Books, 1992.

————. *7 Weeks to Emotional Healing.* New York: Ballantine, 1999.

Libby, A., and I. Stone. "The Hypoascorbemia-Kwashiorkor Approach to Drug Addiction Therapy: A Pilot Study." *J Orthomolecular Psych* 6:4 (1977): 300–308. Available online at: www.seanet.com/~alexs/ ascorbate/197x/libby-af-orthomol_psych-1977-v6-n4-p300.htm.

————. "Letter: Vitamin C and Drug Addiction." *J Orthomolecular Psych* 7:3 (1977): 176. Available online at: www.seanet.com/~alexs/ ascorbate/ 197x/editor-orthomol_psych-1977-v7-n3-p176.htm.

Petralli, G. *Alcoholism: The Cause and the Cure.* Santa Cruz, CA:

Alternative Approaches to End Alcohol Abuse, 2007; www.the101
program.com.

Smith, Lendon. Dr. Smith's bibliography is available at: www.doctor
yourself.com/biblio_lsmith.html.

Werbach, Melvyn, M.D., with Jeffrey Moss, D.D.S. *Textbook of
Nutritional Medicine.* Tarzana, CA: Third Line Press, 1999.

Bibliography

Agnew, N., and A. Hoffer. "Nicotinic Acid Modified Lysergic Acid
Diethylamide Psychosis." *J Mental Sci* 101 (1955): 12–27.

Brody, B. "Guidelines in Treating the Alcoholic Patient in the General Hospital: Orthomolecular Therapy." *J Orthomolecular Psych* 6
(1977): 329–334.

Canner, P.L., K.G. Berge, N.K. Wenger, et al. "Fifteen-year Mortality
in Coronary Drug Project Patients: Long-term Benefit with Niacin." *J
Am College Cardiol* 8 (1986): 1245–1255.

Cheraskin, E., and W.M. Ringsdorf. "A Biochemical Denominator in
the Primary Prevention of Alcoholism." *J Orthomolecular Psych* 9
(1980): 158–163.

Cleary, J. "Treatment of Alcohol Addiction." *J Orthomolecular Med*
2 (1987): 166–168.

Durko, I., E. Papp, I.S. Varga, et al. "Antioxidant Enzyme Levels in
Red Blood Cells of Chronic Alcoholic Men Patients During Oral
Niacin Therapy." *J Orthomolecular Med* 3 (1990): 203–209.

Gentala, E. "The Alcoholic: How Sick into Treatment? How Well
When Discharged?" *J Orthomolecular Psych* 8 (1979): 253–264.

Gesch, C.B., S.M. Hammond, S.E. Hampson, et al. "Influence of
Supplementary Vitamins, Minerals and Essential Fatty Acids on the
Antisocial Behaviour of Young Adult Prisoners. Randomised, Placebo-
controlled Trial." *Br J Psych* 181 (2002): 22–28.

Hartigan, F. *A Biography of Alcoholics Anonymous Cofounder Bill
Wilson.* New York: Thomas Dunne Books/St. Martin's Press, 2000.

Hawkins, D. In: Bill W. (Wilson). "The Vitamin B3 Therapy: A Second Communication to A.A.'s Physicians." February 1968. (Paper was presented at Fordham University Conference on Schizophrenia, January 13, 1968.)

———. In: Hawkins, D., and L. Pauling (eds.). *Orthomolecular Psychiatry,* Section IV. San Francisco: W.H. Freeman, 1973.

———. "Paradigm Blindness: Academic vs. Clinical Medicine." *J Orthomolecular Med* 2006:21: 197–199.

Hoffer, A. "Treatment of Arthritis by Nicotinic Acid and Nicotinamide." *Can Med Assoc J* 81 (1959): 235–238.

———. *Niacin Therapy in Psychiatry.* Springfield, IL: C.C. Thomas, 1962.

———. "Malvaria and the Law." *Psychosomatics* 7 (1966): 303–310.

Hoffer, A., and H. Osmond. *The Hallucinogens.* New York: Academic Press, 1967.

Hoffer, A. "Hong Kong Veterans Study." *J Orthomolecular Psych* 3 (1974): 34–36.

———. "Some Theoretical Principles Basic to Orthomolecular Psychiatric Treatment." In: Hippchen, L.J. (ed.). *Ecologic-Biochemical Approaches to Treatment of Delinquents and Criminals.* New York: Van Nostrand Reinhold, 1978, pp. 31–55.

———. "Behavioral Nutrition." *J Orthomolecular Psych* 8 (1979): 169–175.

———. "Crime, Punishment and Treatment." *J Orthomolecular Psych* 8 (1979): 193–199.

———. "Nutrition and Behavior." In: Bland, J. (ed.). *Medical Applications of Clinical Nutrition.* New Canaan CT: Keats, 1983, pp. 222–251.

———. *Nutritional Therapy: Holistic Approaches to Offender Rehabilitation.* Hippchen, L.J. (ed.). Springfield, IL: C.C. Thomas, 1982, pp. 207–236.

Hoffer, A., and M. Walker. *Putting It All Together: The New Orthomolecular Nutrition.* New Canaan, CT: Keats, 1996.

Hoffer, A. "Treating Children with Learning and/or Behavior Disorders." *Am J Natural Med* 5 (1998): 7–9.

————. *Vitamin B₃ and Schizophrenia: Discovery, Recovery, Controversy.* Kingston, ON, Canada: Quarry Press, 2000.

————. "Negative and Positive Side Effects of Vitamin B₃." *J Orthomolecular Med* 18 (2003): 146–160.

————. *Common Questions on Schizophrenia and Their Answers.* Kingston, ON, Canada: Quarry Press, 1999.

————. *Hoffer's ABC of Natural Nutrition for Children.* Kingston, ON, Canada: Quarry Press, 1999.

————. *Orthomolecular Treatment for Schizophrenia.* New Canaan, CT: Keats, 1999.

————. *Healing Schizophrenia.* Toronto, ON, Canada: CCNM Press, 2004.

————. *Healing Children's Attention and Behavior Disorders.* Toronto, ON, Canada: CCNM Press, 2005.

Hoffer, A., and Andrew W. Saul. *Orthomolecular Medicine for Everyone.* Laguna Beach, CA: Basic Health, 2008.

Jonas, W.B., C.P. Rapoza, and W.F. Blair. "The Effect of Niacinamide on Osteoarthritis: A Pilot Study." *Inflamm Res* 45 (1996): 330–334.

Kahan, F.H. *New Hope for Alcoholics.* New Hyde Park, NY: University Books, 1968.

Kaufman, W. *Common Forms of Niacinamide Deficiency Disease: Aniacin Amidosis.* New Haven, CT: Yale University Press, 1943.

————. *The Common Form of Joint Dysfunction: Its Incidence and Treatment.* Brattleboro, CT: E.L. Hildreth, 1949.

Larson, Joan Mathews. *Alcoholism: The Biochemical Connection.* New York: Villard, 1992.

————. *Seven Weeks to Sobriety.* New York: Fawcett Books, 1997.

Libby, A.F., C.R. Starling, D.K. MacMurray, et al. "Abnormal Blood and Urine Chemistries in an Alcohol and Drug Population: Dramatic Reversals Obtained Quickly from Potentially Serious Diseases." *J Orthomolecular Psych* 11 (1982): 156–181

Libby, A.E., O. Rasmussen, W. Smart, et al. "Methodology: Use of Orthomolecular Techniques for Alcohol and Drug Abuse in a Postdetox Setting." *J Orthomolecular Psych* 11 (1982): 277–288

McCracken, R.D. *Niacin and Human Health Disorders.* Fort Collins, CO: Hygea, 1994.

Pauling, Linus. *How to Live Longer and Feel Better.* New York: W.H. Freeman, 1986.

Reed, B. *Food, Teens and Behavior.* Manitowoc, WI: Natural Press, 1983.

Repogle, W.H., and F.J. Eicke. "Megavitamin Therapy in the Reduction of Anxiety and Depression among Alcoholics." *J Orthomolecular Med* 4 (1989): 221–224.

Schauss, A.G., and C.E. Simonsen. "A Critical Analysis of the Diets of Chronic Juvenile Offenders (Part 1)." *J Orthomolecular Psych* 8 (1979): 149–157.

Schauss, A.G., J. Bland, and C.E. Simonsen. "A Critical Analysis of the Diets of Chronic Juvenile Offenders (Part 2)." *J Orthomolecular Psych* 8 (1979): 222–226.

Simpson, L.O. "Myalgic Encephalomyelitis (ME): A Haemorheological Disorder Manifested as Impaired Capillary Blood Flow." *J Orthomolecular Med* 12 (1997): 69–76.

———. "Omega-3 Fatty Acids and Blood Rheology." *BMJ Rapid Response Section* (March 27, 2006).

Simpson, L.O., and G.P. Herbison. "The Results from Red Cell Shape Analyses of Blood Samples from Members of Myalgic Encephalomyelitis Organizations in Four Countries." *J Orthomolecular Med* 12 (1997): 221–226.

Simpson, L.O., and D.J. O'Neill. "Red Blood Cell Shape, Symptoms and Reportedly Helpful Treatments in Americans with Chronic Disorders." *J Orthomolecular Med* 16 (2001): 157–165.

Smith, R.F. "A Five-year Field Trial of Massive Nicotinic Acid Therapy of Alcoholics in Michigan." *J Orthomolecular Psych* 3 (1974): 327–331.

———. "Status Report Concerning the Use of Megadose Nicotinic Acid in Alcoholics." *J Orthomolecular Psych* 7:1 (1978).

———. *Diagnosis and Treatment of Alcoholism: Ecologic-Biochemical Approaches to Treatment of Delinquents and Criminals.* Hippchen, L.J. (ed.). New York: Van Nostrand Reinhold, 1978, p. 284.

Visscher, M. "You Do What You Eat." *Ode Magazine* (September 8, 2005).

Wilson, Bill ("Bill W.") "The Vitamin B$_3$ Therapy: Communication to AA's Physicians." (The first communication in 1965, the second in 1968, and the third in 1971.) These three out-of-print publications can sometimes be located by an Internet search.

Wittenborn, J.R. "A Search for Responders to Niacin Supplements." *Arch Gen Psych* 31 (1974): 547–552.

REFERENCES

Chapter 1: Nutritional Factors for Alcoholism

1. New York State Office of Alcoholism and Substance Abuse Services. *OASAS Today* 1:1 (September–October 1992).

2. *Health: United States, 2007,* Table 68. Hyattsville, MD: National Center for Health Statistics, 2007.

3. Ibid.

4. *Deaths: Final Data for 2004,* Tables 10, 23. Hyattsville, MD: National Center for Health Statistics, 2005.

5. Ibid.

6. Ray, O., and C. Ksir. *Drugs, Society and Human Behavior.* St. Louis: Mosby, 1990, p. 173.

7. Kessler, R.C., P.A. Berglund, O. Demler, et al. "Lifetime Prevalence and Age-of-onset Distributions of DSM-IV Disorders in the National Comorbidity Survey Replication (NCS-R)." *Arch Gen Psych* 62:6 (June 2005): 593–602.

8. Pauling, L. *How to Live Longer and Feel Better,* Revised ed. Corvallis, OR: Oregon State University Press, 2006, p. 93.

Chapter 2: What Causes Addictions?

1. New York State Office of Alcoholism and Substance Abuse Services. *OASAS Today* 1:1 (September–October 1992).

2. Center for Science in the Public Interest. *Liquid Candy: How Soft Drinks Are Harming Americans' Health.* Available online at: www.cspinet.org/liquid candy/index.html.

Chapter 3: Niacin for Alcoholism: How It All Began

1. Armstrong, R.W., and J. Gould. "The Nature and Treatment of Delirium Tremens and Allied Conditions." *J Mental Sci* 101:422 (January 1955): 70–84. Gould, J. "Treatment of Delirium, Psychosis, and Coma Due to Drugs." *Lancet* 1:6760 (March 1953): 570–573.

2. Kaufman, W. *The Common Form of Niacinamide Deficiency Disease: Aniacinamidosis.* New Haven, CT: Yale University Press, 1943. Kaufman, W. *The Common Form of Joint Dysfunction: Its Incidence and Treatment.* Brattleboro, VT: E.L. Hildreth, 1949. Both available online at: www.doctoryourself.com.

Chapter 4: Conquering Alcoholism Nutritionally

1. Glória, L., M. Cravo, M.E. Camilo, et al. "Nutritional Deficiencies in Chronic Alcoholics: Relation to Dietary Intake and Alcohol Consumption." *Am J Gastroenterol* 92:3 (March 1997): 485–489.

2. Glória, L., M. Cravo, M.E. Camilo, et al. "Nutritional Deficiencies in Chronic Alcoholics: Relation to Dietary Intake and Alcohol Consumption." *Am J Gastroenterol* 92:3 (March 1997): 485–489. Majumdar, S.K., G.K. Shaw, A.D. Thomson. "Vitamin Utilization Status in Chronic Alcoholics." *Intl J Vitamin Nutr Res* 51:1 (1981): 54–58.

3. Baker, H. "A Vitamin Profile of Alcoholism." *Intl J Vitamin Nutr Res Suppl* 24 (1983): 179–184. Majumdar, S.K., G.K. Shaw, P. O'Gorman, et al. "Blood Vitamin Status (B_1, B_2, B_6, folic acid and B_{12}) in Patients with Alcoholic Liver Disease." *Intl J Vitamin Nutr Res* 52:3 (1982): 266–271.

4. Ostrovski S.I., and V.P. Grinevich. "Effect of Supplementary Vitamin Administration on Free Amino Acids in the Liver and Brain of Rats with Alcoholic Intoxication." *Vopr Pitan* 3 (May-June 1988): 41–45.

5. Ryle, P.R., and A.D. Thomson. "Nutrition and Vitamins in Alcoholism." *Contemp Issues Clin Biochem* 1 (1984): 188–224.

6. Boggs, W. *Arch Dis Childhood* (June 2004).

7. Poulos, C. Jean, Sc.D., Ph.D. "What Effects Do Corrective Nutritional Practices Have on Alcoholics?" *J Orthomolecular Psych* 10:1 (1981): 61–64.

8. Gerson, Charlotte, and Morton Walker, DPM. *The Gerson Therapy.* New York: Kensington, 2001. Gerson, Charlotte, with Beata Bishop. *Healing the Gerson Way: Defeating Cancer and Other Chronic Diseases.* Carmel Valley, CA: Totality Books, 2007.

9. Smith, R.F. "Status Report Concerning the Use of Megadose Niacin in Alcoholics." *J Orthomolecular Med* 7:1 (1978): 52–55.

10. Cleary, John P., M.D. "Etiology and Biological Treatment of Alcohol Addiction." *J Orthomolecular Med* 2:3 (1987): 166–168.

11. Hoffer, A., and H. Osmond. "Concerning an Etiological Factor in Alcoholism. The Possible Role of Adrenochrome Metabolism." *Qtr J Stud Alcohol* 20 (1959): 750–756.

12. Rizakallah, G.S., M.K. Mertens, M.L. Brown, et al. "Clinical Inquiries: Should Liver Enzymes be Checked in a Patient Taking Niacin?" *J Fam Pract* 54:3 (March 2005): 265–268. Litin, S.C., and C.F. Anderson. "Nicotinic Acid-associated Myopathy: A Report of Three Cases." *Am J Med* 86:4 (April 1989): 481–483. Goldstein, M.R. "Nicotinic Acid-associated Myopathy." *Am J Med* 87:2 (August 1989): 248. Alderman, J.D., R.C. Pasternak, F.M. Sacks, et al. "Effect of a Modified, Well-tolerated Niacin Regimen on Serum Total Cholesterol, High-density Lipoprotein Cholesterol and the Cholesterol to High-density Lipoprotein Ratio." *Am J Cardiol* 64:12 (October 1989): 725–729.

13. Guyton, J.R., and H.E. Bays. "Safety Considerations with Niacin Therapy." *Am J Cardiol* 99:6A (March 2007): 22C–31C.

14. Fonda, M.L. "Vitamin B_6 Metabolism and Binding to Proteins in the Blood of Alcoholic and Nonalcoholic Men." *Alcohol Clin Exp Res* 17:6 (December 1993): 1171–1178. Fonda, M.L., S.G. Brown, M.W. Pendleton. "Concentration of Vitamin B_6 and Activities of Enzymes of B_6 Metabolism in the Blood of Alcoholic and Nonalcoholic Men." *Alcohol Clin Exp Res* 13:6 (December 1989): 804–809.

15. Bonjour, J.P. "Vitamins and Alcoholism. III. Vitamin B_6." *Intl J Vitamin Nutr Res* 50:2 (1980): 215–230. Parker, T.H., J.P. Marshall, 2nd, R.K. Roberts, et al. "Effect of Acute Alcohol Ingestion on Plasma Pyridoxal 5'-Phosphate." *Am J Clin Nutr* 32:6 (June 1979): 1246–1252.

16. Lorentzen, H.F., A.M. Fugleholm, K. Weismann. "Zinc Deficien-

cy and Pellagra in Alcohol Abuse." *Ugeskr Laeger* 162:50 (December 2000): 6854–6856. Jendryczko, A., and M. Drózdz. "Alcoholism-induced Zinc Deficiency in Mother and Fetus." *Wiad Lek* 42:19–21 (October/November 1989): 1052–1054. Skal'ny, A.V., and A.M. Skosyreva. "Zinc Deficiency in the Mother, Fetus and Progeny in Alcohol Abuse." *Akush Ginekol (Mosk)* 4 (April 1987): 6–8.

17. Bovt, V.D., V.A. Ieshchenko, M.M. Mal'ko, et al. "Study on the Connection of Alcohol Motivation with Zinc Content Changes in the Hippocampus." *Fiziol Zh* 47:3 (2001): 54–57.

18. Skal'ny, A.V., E.N. Kukhtina, I.P. Ol'khovskaia, et al. "Reduction of Voluntary Alcohol Consumption Under the Effects of Prolonged-action Zinc." *Biull Eksp Biol Med* 113:4 (April 1992): 383–385.

19. Proskuriakova, T.V., V.M. Gurtovenko, E.P. Gorshkova. "The Evaluation of the Effect of Zinc Sulfate on Primary Immune Response Indices Under Alcoholic Intoxication." *Eksp Klin Farmakol* 59:2 (March-April 1996): 47–49.

20. Caballería, J., A. Giménez, H. Andreu, et al. "Zinc Administration Improves Gastric Alcohol Dehydrogenase Activity and First-pass Metabolism of Ethanol in Alcohol-fed Rats." *Alcohol Clin Exp Res* 21:9 (December 1997): 1619–1622.

21. Replogle, W.H., and F.J. Eicke. "Megavitamin Therapy in the Reduction of Anxiety and Depression Among Alcoholics." *J Orthomolecular Med* 4:4 (1989): 221–224.

22. Manzardo, A.M., E.C. Penick, J. Knop, et al. "Neonatal Vitamin K Might Reduce Vulnerability to Alcohol Dependence in Danish Men." *J Stud Alcohol* 66:5 (September 2005): 586–592.

23. Coppen, A., and C. Bolander-Gouaille. "Treatment of Depression: Time to Consider Folic Acid and Vitamin B12." *J Psychopharmacol* 19:1 (January 2005): 59–65. Also: Merry, J., M. Abou-Saleh, A. Coppen. "Alcoholism, Depression and Plasma Folate." *Br J Psych* 141 (July 1982): 103–104.

24. Delgado-Sanchez, L., D. Godkar, S. Niranjan. "Pellagra: Rekindling of an Old Flame." *Am J Ther* 15:2 (March-April 2008): 173–175.

25. Cox, F.M., J.H. Cornel, M. Aramideh. "A Man with the Combination of Dry and Wet Beriberi." *Ned Tijdschr Geneeskd* 150:24 (June 2006): 1347–1350.

26. Bohrer, I., M. Roy, W. Nager, et al. "Scurvy—A Wrongly Forgotten Avitaminosis." *MMW Fortschr Med* 149:45 (November 2007): 41–43.

27. Smets, Y.F., N. Bokani, P.H. de Meijer, et al. "Tetany Due to Excessive Use of Alcohol: A Possible Magnesium Deficiency." *Ned Tijdschr Geneeskd* 148:14 (April 2004): 641–644.

28. Olszynski, W.P., K. Shawn Davison, J.D. Adachi, et al. "Osteoporosis in Men: Epidemiology, Diagnosis, Prevention, and Treatment." *Clin Ther* 26:1 (January 2004): 15–28.

29. Thomson, A.D. "Mechanisms of Vitamin Deficiency in Chronic Alcohol Misusers and the Development of the Wernicke-Korsakoff Syndrome." *Alcohol (Suppl)* 35:1 (May-June 2000): 2–7.

30. Gueguen, S., P. Pirollet, P. Leroy, et al. "Changes in Serum Retinol, Alpha-tocopherol, Vitamin C, Carotenoids, Zinc and Selenium after Micronutrient Supplementation during Alcohol Rehabilitation." *J Am Coll Nutr* 22:4 (August 2003): 303–310.

31. For further information on alcohol, depression, and anxiety, see: Prousky, Jonathan. *Anxiety: Orthomolecular Diagnosis and Treatment.* Toronto, ON, Canada: CCNM Press, 2006. Challem, Jack. *The Food-Mood Solution: All-Natural Ways to Banish Anxiety, Depression, Anger, Stress, Overeating, and Alcohol and Drug Problems—and Feel Good Again.* New York: Wiley, 2008.

32. Hoes, M.J.AJ.M., M.D. "Psychiatric Significance of the Plasma Concentrations of Magnesium and Vitamin B_1 in Alcoholism and Delirium Tremens: Alcohol is a Biological Solvent." *Orthomolecular Psych* 10:3 (1981): 159–165.

33. Smith, L. H. (ed.). *Clinical Guide to the Use of Vitamin C.* Tacoma, WA: Life Sciences Press, 1988.

34. Levy, Thomas E., M.D., J.D. *Vitamin C, Infectious Diseases, and Toxins: Curing the Incurable.* Philadelphia: Xlibris, 2002.

35. Susick, R.L., Jr., G.D. Abrams, C.A. Zurawski, et al. "Ascorbic Acid Chronic Alcohol Consumption in the Guinea Pig." *Toxicol Appl Pharmacol* 84:2 (June 1986): 329–335. Zannoni, V.G., J.I. Brodfuehrer, R.C. Smart, et al. "Ascorbic Acid, Alcohol, and Environmental Chemicals." *Ann NY Acad Sci* 498 (1987): 364–388. Susick, R.L., Jr., and V.G. Zannoni. "Ascorbic Acid and Alcohol Oxidation." *Biochem Pharmacol* 33:24 (December 1984): 3963–3969.

36. Horrobin, D.F. "A Biochemical Basis for Alcoholism and Alcohol-induced Damage Including the Fetal Alcohol Syndrome and Cirrhosis: Interference with Essential Fatty Acid and Prostaglandin Metabolism." *Med Hypotheses* 6:9 (September 1980): 929–942. Horrobin, D.F. "Essential Fatty Acids, Prostaglandins, and Alcoholism: An Overview." *Alcohol Clin Exp Res* 11:1 (February 1987): 2–9. Wolkin, A., D. Segarnick, J. Sierkierski, et al. "Essential Fatty Acid Supplementation During Early Alcohol Abstinence." *Alcohol Clin Exp Res* 11:1 (February 1987): 87–92.

37. Segarnick, D.J., D. Mandio Cordasco, V. Agura, et al. "Gamma-linolenic Acid Inhibits the Development of the Ethanol-induced Fatty Liver." *Prostaglandins Leukot Med* 17:3 (March 1985): 277–282.

38. Rogers, L.L., R.B. Pelton, R.J. Williams. "Voluntary Alcohol Consumption by Rats Following Administration of Glutamine." *J Biol Chem* 214:2 (June 1955): 503–506. Rogers, L.L., and R.B. Pelton. "Glutamine in the Treatment of Alcoholism: A Preliminary Report." *Qtr J Stud Alcohol* 18:4 (December 1957): 581–587.

39. Bobrova, N.P., V.G. Koval'chuk, O.V. Chumakova. "Effect of Chronic Alcohol Intoxication, Termination of Ethanol Administration, and Treatment of Abstinence with Glutamine and Riboflavin on Neuromediatory Systems of Gamma-aminobutyric Acid and Acetylcholine in the Rat Brain." *Vopr Med Khim* 28:1 (January-February 1982): 103–106. Garbin, O., and V. Vartanian. "Habit or Addiction: Observations After Treatment of Alcoholics with L-glutamine." *Clin Ter* 51:4 (November 1969): 367–371. Garbin, O., and V. Vartanian. "Treatment of Alcoholism with Parenteral Administration of L-glutamine." *Minerva Med* 59:80 (October 1968): 4254–4261. Stolt, G. "Glutamine in the Treatment of Alcoholic Intoxication. A Double-blind Trial." *Nord Psykiatr Tidsskr* 22:1 (1968): 39–43.

40. Ussher, M., A.K. Sampuran, R. Doshi, et al. "Acute Effect of a Brief Bout of Exercise on Alcohol Urges." *Addiction* 99:12 (December 2004): 1542–1547. Ermalinski, R., P.G. Hanson, B. Lubin, et al. "Impact of a Body-Mind Treatment Component on Alcoholic Inpatients." *J Psychosoc Nurs Mental Health Serv* 35:7 (July 1997): 39–45.

41. Gelderloos, P., K.G. Walton, D.W. Orme-Johnson, et al. "Effectiveness of the Transcendental Meditation Program in Preventing and Treating Substance Misuse: A Review." *Intl J Addictions* 26:3 (1991): 293–325. Alexander, C.N., P. Robinson, M. Rainforth. "Treating and

Preventing Alcohol, Nicotine, and Drug Abuse through Transcendental Meditation: A Review and Statistical Meta-analysis." *Alcoholism Treat Qtr* 11:1-2 (1994): 13–87. Taub, E., S.S. Steiner, E. Weingarten, et al. "Effectiveness of Broad-spectrum Approaches to Relapse Prevention in Severe Alcoholism: A Long-term, Randomised, Controlled Trial of Transcendental Meditation, EMG Biofeedback and Electronic Neurotherapy." *Alcoholism Treat Qtr* 11:1–2 (1994): 187–220. Bleick, C.R. "Case Histories: Using the Transcendental Meditation Program with Alcoholics and Addicts." *Alcoholism Treat Qtr* 11:3–4 (1994): 243–269. Shafii, M., R.A. Lavely, R.D. Jaffe. "Meditation and the Prevention of Alcohol Abuse." *Am J Psych* 132 (1974): 942–945.

Chapter 5: Results of Vitamin Treatment

1. Hartigan, Francis. *Bill W.: A Biography of Alcoholics Anonymous Cofounder Bill Wilson.* New York: St. Martin's Griffin, 2001.

2. Cleary, John P. "Etiology and Biological Treatment of Alcohol Addiction." *J Orthomolecular Med* 2:3 (1987). Vitale, J.J., D.M. Hegsted, H. McGrath, et al. "The Effect of Acetate, Pyruvate, and Glucose on Alcohol Metabolism." *J Biol Chem* 210:2 (1954): 753–759. Available online at: www.jbc.org/cgi/reprint/210/2/753.pdf.

3. Beasley, Joseph D., M.D. www.addictionend.org.

4. Hoffer, A. "Malvaria, Schizophrenia and the HOD Test." *Intl J Neuropsych* 2 (1965): 175–177. Kelm, H., A. Hoffer, R.W. Hall. "Reliability of the Hoffer-Osmond Diagnostic Test." *J Clin Psych* 23 (1967): 380–382. Kelm, H., M.J. Callbeck, A. Hoffer. "A Short Form of the Hoffer-Osmond Diagnostic Test." *Intl J Neuropsych* 3 (1967): 489–490. Kelm, H. "Hoffer-Osmond Diagnostic Test: A Review." *J Schizophrenia* 1 (2nd Quarter 1967): 90. Kelm, H., and A. Kelm. "A Further Study of the Validity of the Hoffer-Osmond Diagnostic Test." *J Orthomolecular Med* 4 (4th Quarter 1989): 225.

5. Wittenborn, J.R. "A Search for Responders to Niacin Supplements." *Arch Gen Psych* 31 (1974): 547–552.

Chapter 6: The Controversy Over Psychedelic Therapy

1. Mangini, M. "Treatment of Alcoholism Using Psychedelic Drugs: A Review of the Program of Research." *J Psychoactive Drugs* 30:4 (October–December 1998): 381–418.

2. Sigafoos, J., V.A. Green, C. Edrisinha, et al. "Flashback to the 1960s: LSD in the Treatment of Autism." *Dev Neurorehabil* 10:1 (January-March 2007): 75–81.

3. Delgado, P.L., and F.A. Moreno. "Hallucinogens, Serotonin and Obsessive-compulsive Disorder." *J Psychoactive Drugs* 30:4 (October-December 1998): 359–366. Moreno, F.A., C.B. Wiegand, E.K. Taitano, et al. "Safety, Tolerability, and Efficacy of Psilocybin in 9 Patients with Obsessive-compulsive Disorder." *J Clin Psych* 67:11 (November 2006): 1735–1740.

4. Riedlinger, T.J., and J.E. Riedlinger. "Psychedelic and Entactogenic Drugs in the Treatment of Depression." *J Psychoactive Drugs* 26:1 (January-March 1994): 41–55.

Chapter 7: Stopping Tobacco Smoking and Caffeine Use

1. *Drug Alcohol Dependence* 337 (1993): 211–213.

2. Ibid.

3. Clarkes, R. "Niacin for Nicotine?" *Lancet* 1:8174 (1980): 936.

4. Prousky, J.E. "Vitamin B₃ for Nicotine Addiction." *J Orthomolecular Med* 18 (2003): 56–57. By permission.

5. Cleary, J.P. "The NAD Deficiency Diseases." *J Orthomolecular Med* 1:3 (1986): 149–157. Cleary, J.P. "Etiology and Biological Treatment of Alcohol Addiction." *J Orthomolecular Med* 2:3 (1987): 166–168.

6. Cleary, J.P. "Etiology and Biological Treatment of Alcohol Addiction." *J Orthomolecular Med* 2:3 (1987): 166–168.

7. Patrick, L. "The Biochemistry and Pathology of Nicotine Dependence." *J Naturopath Med* 8:2 (1998): 45–48.

8. Cheraskin, E., W.M. Ringsdorf, Jr., A.T. Setyaadmadja, et al. "Effect of Caffeine versus Placebo Supplementation on Blood-glucose Concentration." *Lancet* 1:7503 (June 1967): 1299–1300. Cheraskin, E., W.M. Ringsdorf, Jr. "Blood-glucose Levels after Caffeine." *Lancet* 2:7569 (September 1968): 689.

9. Carper, J. "Your Food Pharmacy." Syndicated column (June 15, 1994).

10. Center for Science in the Public Interest. *Liquid Candy: How Soft Drinks Are Harming Americans' Health*. Available online at: www.cspinet.org/liquidcandy/index.html.

11. Wilcox, A, C. Weinberg, D. Baird. "Caffeinated Beverages and Decreased Fertility." *Lancet* 2:8626-7 (December 1988): 1473–1476.

12. Whalen, Ruth. *Welcome to the Dance: Caffeine Allergy—A Masked Cerebral Allergy and Progressive Toxic Dementia*. Victoria, BC, Canada: Trafford Publishing, 2005.

13. Cameron, Ewan, M.D., and Linus Pauling. *Cancer and Vitamin C*. Philadelphia: Camino Books, 1993, p. xii.

14. Clarke, John H. *The Prescriber*, 9th edition. Essex, England: C.W. Daniel, 1972.

Chapter 8: Orthomolecular Support During Withdrawal and Drug Overdose

1. Libby, Alfred F., and Irwin Stone. "The Hypoascorbemia-Kwashiorkor Approach to Drug Addiction Therapy: A Pilot Study." *J Orthomolecular Psych* 6:4 (1977): 300–308.

2. Cathcart, R.F. "Vitamin C, Titration to Bowel Tolerance, Anascorbemia, and Acute Induced Scurvy." *Med Hypothesis* 7 (1981): 1359–1376. Cathcart, R.F. "A Unique Function for Ascorbate." *Med Hypothesis* 35 (May 1991): 32–37. Cathcart, R.F. "The Third Face of Vitamin C." *J Orthomolecular Med* 7:4 (1993): 197–200.

3. Evangelou, A., V. Kalfakakou, P. Georgakas, et al. "Ascorbic Acid (Vitamin C) Effects on Withdrawal Syndrome of Heroin Abusers." *In Vivo* 14:2 (March-April 2000): 363–366.

4. Levy, Thomas E., M.D. *Vitamin C, Infectious Diseases, and Toxins: Curing the Incurable*. Philadelphia: Xlibris, 2002.

5. Cameron, Ewan, M.D., and Linus Pauling. *Cancer and Vitamin C*. Philadelphia: Camino Books, 1993, p. xii.

INDEX

ABOUT THE AUTHORS

Born on a Saskatchewan farm in 1917, **Abram Hoffer** graduated with a B.S. in agriculture from the University of Saskatchewan in 1938. He also has a master's degree in agricultural chemistry and a Ph.D. in biochemistry. He got his M.D. from the University of Toronto in 1949 and completed psychiatric training in 1954. His early work led to the use of vitamin B_3 in treating schizophrenia and other psychiatric conditions, and he demonstrated the effectiveness of niacin as an anticholesterol treatment. Dr. Hoffer was involved in the formation of the *Journal of Orthomolecular Medicine* and has published over 600 reports and articles, as well as 30 books. Recently, he was awarded the Dr. Rogers Prize for his contribution to alternative and complementary medicine.

Andrew W. Saul has over 30 years of experience in natural health education and has taught nutrition, health science, and cell biology at the college level for nine years. He is editor of the Orthomolecular Medicine News Service and assistant editor of the *Journal of Orthomolecular Medicine*. He is the author of *Doctor Yourself: Natural Healing That Works* and *Fire Your Doctor! How to Be Independently Healthy*. He is also coauthor, with Dr. Abram Hoffer, of *Orthomolecular Medicine for Everyone*, and, with Dr. Steve Hickey, of *Vitamin C: The Real Story*. (All four books are available from Basic Health Publications.) His popular peer-reviewed, noncommercial natural healing website is www.DoctorYourself.com.